Obsessive Compulsive Disorder:

A Practical Guide

Obsessive Compulsive Disorder:

A Practical Guide

Naomi Fineberg MA(Cantab), MBBS MRCPsych
Consultant Psychiatrist
East and North Herts Specialist OCD Service
Queen Elizabeth II Hospital
Howlands
Welwyn Garden City
Herts, UK

Donatella Marazziti MD
Psychiatrist
Department of Psychiatry, Neurobiology, Pharmacology and
Biotechnology
University of Pisa
Pisa, Italy

Dan J Stein BSc (Med), MBChB, FRCPC
Director
MRC Unit on Anxiety Disorders
Department of Psychiatry
University of Stellenbosch
Cape Town
South Africa
and Department of Psychiatry
University of Florida
Gainesville FL, USA

Martin Dunitz

Cover illustration designed and drawn by Marrianne Behm

© 2001 Martin Dunitz Ltd, a member of the Taylor & Francis group

First published in the United Kingdom in 2001
by Martin Dunitz Ltd, The Livery House, 7–9 Pratt Street, London NW1 0AE

Tel.:   +44 (0) 20 74822202
Fax.:   +44 (0) 20 72670159
E-mail: info.dunitz@tandf.co.uk
Website: http://www.dunitz.co.uk

A CIP record for this book is available from the British Library.

ISBN 1 85317 919 1

Distributed in the USA by
Fulfilment Center
Taylor & Francis
7625 Empire Drive
Florence, KY 41042, USA
Toll Free Tel: 1-800-634-7064
Email: cserve@routledge_ny.com

Distributed in Canada by
Taylor & Francis
74 Rolark Drive
Scarborough
Ontario M1R G2, Canada
Toll Free Tel: 1-877-226-2237
Email: tal_fran@istar.ca

Distributed in the rest of the world by
ITPS Limited
Cheriton House
North Way, Andover
Hampshire SP10 5BE, UK
Tel: +44 (0)1264 332424
Email: reception@itps.co.uk

Composition by Wearset, Boldon, Tyne and Wear

Printed and bound in Great Britain by Biddles Ltd, Guildford and King's Lynn.

Contents

Dedication

In memory of Sidney Fineberg, and with grateful thanks to my mentors, Barry Everitt, Stuart Montgomery and Philip Cowen, my patients and my husband, Edwin.

Naomi Fineberg

I dedicate this book to OCD patients who inspired and continue to sustain my interest in their sufference; to my mentor, Professor Giovanni B Cassano, who shaped and oriented my professional life; and to our editor and friend, Mrs Ruth Dunitz, who enthusiastically shared with us the 'adventure' of developing this book.

Donatella Marazziti

For Heather, Gabriella and Joshua, and with gratitude to the people with OCD who have contributed their knowledge and time to the research efforts of the MRC Unit on Anxiety Disorders.

Dan J Stein

Contributors

Andreas Broocks MD, PhD
Medical University of Lübeck
Clinic for Psychiatry and
Psychotherapy
Ratzeburger Allee 160
23538 Lübeck
Germany

David Cohen MD
CNRS UMR 7593
Hôpital La Salpêtrière
Pavillon Clérambault
47 boulevard de l'Hôpital
75013 Paris
France

Peter Farvolden PhD
Centre for Addiction and Mental Health
33 Russell Street
Toronto, ON, M5S 2S1
Canada

Naomi A Fineberg MA(Cantab), MBBS
MRCPsych
East and North Herts Specialist OCD
Service
Queen Elizabeth II Hospital
Howlands
Welwyn Garden City
Herts, AL7 4HQ
UK

Martine F Flament MD, PhD
CNRS UMR 7593
Hôpital La Salpêtrière
Pavillon Clérambault
47 boulevard de l'Hôpital
75013 Paris
France

Toby D Goldsmith MD
University of Florida, College of
Medicine
Department of Psychiatry
PO Box 100256
Gainesville FL 32610-0256
USA

Wayne K Goodman MD
University of Florida, College of
Medicine
Department of Psychiatry
PO Box 100256
Gainesville FL 32610-0256
USA

Brian Harvey BPharm, BPharm (Hons),
MPharm, PhD
Department of Pharmacology
University of Potschefstroom
Potschefstroom
South Africa

Fritz Hohagen MD, PhD
Medical University of Lübeck
Clinic for Psychiatry and
Psychotherapy
Ratzeburger Allee 160
23538 Lübeck
Germany

Lorrin M Koran MD
Department of Psychiatry and
Behavioral Sciences
and OCD Clinic, Room 2363
Stanford University Medical Center
401 Quarry Road
Stanford, CA 94305-5721
USA

James V Lucey MD, PhD, MRCPsych, FRCPI
Royal College of Surgeons in Ireland
Department of Psychiatry
Academic Centre, James Connolly
Memorial Hospital
Dublin 15
Ireland

Christopher J McDougle MD
Department of Psychiatry
Indiana University School of Medicine
Clinical Building, room 299
541 Clinical Drive
Indianapolis, IN 46202
USA

Catherine Mancini MD
Department of Psychiatry and
Behavioural Neurosciences
McMaster University
Anxiety Disorders Clinic
Hamilton Health Sciences Corporation
McMaster University Medical Centre
1200 Main Street West
Hamilton, ON, L8N 3Z5
Canada

Donatella Marazziti MD
Department of Psychiatry,
Neurobiology, Pharmacology and
Biotechnology
University of Pisa
Via Roma, 67
56100 Pisa
Italy

Jonathan M Oakman PhD
Department of Psychology
University of Waterloo
Waterloo, ON, N2L 3G1
Canada

David L Pauls PhD
Child Study Center and Department of
Psychology
Yale University School of Medicine
333 Cedar Street
New Haven CT 06510
USA

Ann Roberts MA(Cantab), MBBS MRCGP
MRCPsych
East and North Herts Specialist OCD
Service
Queen Elizabeth II Hospital
Howlands
Welwyn Garden City
Herts, AL7 4HQ
UK

Soraya Seedat MBChB, MMed (Psych)
MRC Unit of Anxiety Disorders
Department of Psychiatry
University of Stellenbosch
Cape Town
South Africa

Nathan A Shapira MD
University of Florida, College of
Medicine
Department of Psychiatry
PO Box 100256
Gainesville FL 32610-0256
USA

Dan J Stein BSc (Med), MBChB, FRCPC
MRC Unit of Anxiety Disorders
Department of Psychiatry
University of Stellenbosch
Cape Town
South Africa
and Department of Psychiatry
University of Florida
Gainesville FL
USA

Frederick Toates Dphil, DSc
Department of Biological Sciences
The Open University
Milton Keynes
MK7 6AA
UK

Michael Van Ameringen MD
Department of Psychiatry and
Behavioural Neurosciences
McMaster University
Anxiety Disorders Clinic
Hamilton Health Sciences Corporation
McMaster University Medical Centre
1200 Main Street West
Hamilton, ON, L8N 3Z5
Canada

Kelda H Walsh MD
Department of Psychiatry
Indiana University School of Medicine
Riley Hospital for Children
702 Barnhill Drive, room 3701
Indianapolis, IN 46202
USA

Joseph Zohar MD
Chaim Sheba Medical Center
Division of Psychiatry
Tel-Hashomer 52621
Israel

Preface

Obsessive compulsive disorder is now recognized as one of the most common psychiatric disorders, and as the tenth most disabling of all medical disorders. Fortunately, major advances in our understanding of its neurobiological basis and the discovery of robust treatments offer new hope for people with OCD.

Nevertheless, despite the increased recognition of the prevalence and morbidity of OCD, and the introduction of effective treatments, people with OCD continue to remain underdiagnosed and inappropriately treated. It is important for specialist clinicians to be able to educate the public about this disorder, and to provide primary care colleagues with up-to-date information.

In this volume, we attempt to provide a practical guide to the diagnosis, assessment, and management of OCD. Summaries of exciting discoveries in the psychobiology of OCD are included, and pathways for future research considered. This is a book by and for clinicians, and we hope that it will prove useful in clinical settings.

We would like to thank Ruth Dunitz for encouraging and guiding this project.

NF, DM, DJS

1

Obsessive compulsive disorder: a twenty-first century perspective

Naomi Fineberg and Ann Roberts

> MACBETH: *How does your patient, doctor?*
> DOCTOR: *Not so sick, my lord,*
> *As she is troubled with thick-coming fancies*
> *That keep her from her rest.*

(From Shakespeare's *Macbeth,* act V scene III; circa 1606)

Throughout history, our conceptualization of obsessive compulsive disorder (OCD) has been changing alongside changes in the way we have viewed the world. With the dawning of the Renaissance in western Europe, religious explanations based on demonic possession were superseded by a more humanistic understanding. By the early seventeenth century, the obsessions that drove Shakespeare's Lady Macbeth to suicide were recognized to be a product of her guilty mind, for which there was no medical cure.

Obsessions and compulsions were first described in the medical literature of the early nineteenth century. They were viewed as an unusual expression of melancholia. By the beginning of the twentieth century, with the development of psychoanalysis, the focus shifted onto psychological explanations based on unconscious conflicts, but this did not provide a useful strategy for treatment. The subsequent application of learning theory to OCD led to the development of effective behavioural treatments in the 1960s and 1970s.

Compared with the pace of these historical developments, modern understanding of OCD has expanded with dramatic speed. The development of effective medical treatments of OCD has revolutionized the outlook for sufferers and propelled OCD to the forefront of scientific attention. With the growth of research into the epidemiology, psychopharmacology, neurobiology, neuropsychology and genetics of OCD, reviewed throughout this publication, the emphasis has once again swung back toward a medical model. As we enter the twenty-first century, we now recognize OCD as a common, treatable form of major mental disorder.

Diagnostic classification

Both the World Health Organization's International Classification of Diseases, 10th revision (ICD-10) and the American Psychiatric Association's *Diagnostic and Statistical Manual*, 4th edition (DSM-IV) recognize obsessions and/or compulsions as the core symptoms of OCD.[1,2] Obsessions are defined as unwanted ideas, images or impulses which repeatedly enter the individual's mind. Although recognized as being generated by the individual, they are egodystonic and distressing. Compulsions are repetitive stereotyped behaviours or mental acts that are driven by rules that must be applied rigidly. They are not inherently enjoyable and do not result in the completion of any useful task. They may or may not be linked to underlying obsessional thoughts such as worries about contamination or concerns about harm to others.

In both diagnostic systems either disabling obsessions or compulsions (or both) will satisfy a diagnosis. The ICD-10 applies a more rigorous threshold, requiring the symptoms to be present on most days for a period of at least 2 weeks (Table 1.1). Resistance toward the obsessions or compulsions need not always be present, and in chronic cases patients often find that active resistance makes the symptoms worse.

The DSM-IV has prioritized anxiety as a core symptom, and classifies OCD with the anxiety disorders, even though OCD shares few features with the other disorders in this group. In contrast, the ICD-10 has followed a European tradition in conceptualizing OCD as a 'stand-alone' disorder. In the ICD-10, OCD is placed independently within the category of neurotic, stress-related and somatoform disorders.

Further separation of OCD is likely in the future, informed by the growing clinical and neurobiological findings that place the disorder at the heart of a 'spectrum' of OCD-related disorders including hypochondriasis,

Table 1.1   ICD-10 criteria for OCD.

A	Either obsessions or compulsions (or both) present on most days for a period of at least 2 weeks

B	Obsessions (thoughts, ideas or images) and compulsions share the following features, all of which must be present:
	  acknowledged as originating from the mind of the patient, not from outside
	  repetitive and unpleasant: at least one must be acknowledged as excessive or unreasonable
	  resisted (but if very long-standing, resistance may be minimal); at least one must be unsuccessfully resisted
	  carrying out the obsessive thought or compulsive act is not in itself pleasurable

Adapted from ICD-10.[1] Reproduced with kind permission of the International Council on OCD. Adapted from International Council on OCD, *Update on OCD* (Medical Action Communications, 1995).

body dysmorphic disorder, trichotillomania, tic disorders and depersonalization disorder (see Chapter 3).[3,4]

How common is OCD?

After the pioneering epidemiological catchment area (ECA) studies carried out by the National Institute of Mental Health in the early 1980s reported that the prevalence of OCD was substantially higher than expected,[5,6] repeated population studies using similar methods have demonstrated a lifetime prevalence of 2–3% worldwide.[7] Taiwan and India were the only exceptions, with rates below 1%. If these estimates are accurate, then OCD affects more than 50 million people in the world today. The prevalence does not appear to be influenced by socioeconomic status, educational achievement, or ethnicity. The disorder is more common than schizophrenia, and about half as common as depression (Table 1.2). Yet the illness remains largely under-recognized, and the psychosocial and economic costs to society from untreated OCD are high.[8] It is not surprising that the World Health Organization has now recognized OCD as a public health priority.

While there is little doubt that the 'hidden epidemic' of OCD exists, the actual prevalence of clinically relevant disorder has been called into question. In the ECA studies lay interviewers were trained to make DSM-III diagnoses using the Diagnostic Interview Schedule (DIS).[5,6] However, clinical reappraisal of DIS-positive cases resulted in less than 25% continuing to meet the criteria for OCD.[9,10] One explanation is that the rates of illness reported in the original ECA studies may have been exaggerated. Alternatively, the findings may reflect variability in the severity of the disorder over time. Longitudinal studies in community-based samples

Table 1.2 Prevalence of OCD reported by the NIMH epidemiological catchment area study.

	Prevalence rates	
	Lifetime (%)	6 months (%)
Major depression	5.2	2.9
OCD	**2.5**	**1.6**
Schizophrenia	1.6	0.9
Panic disorder	1.4	0.8
Severe cognitive impairment	1.2	1.2
Anorexia nervosa	0.1	–

In: Robins et al (1984).[5] Reproduced with kind permission of the International Council on OCD. Adapted from International Council on OCD, *Update on OCD* (Medical Action Communications: Egham, Surrey, UK 1995).

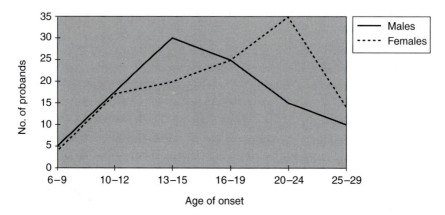

Figure 1.1

Age at onset of OCD. Adapted with permission from Rasmussen SA, Eisen JL. Epidemiology of obsessive compulsive disorder. *J Clin Psychiatry* (1990); **51**: 10–13.[14] Copyright 1990 Physicians Postgraduate Press. Reprinted by permission.

have shown that the condition fluctuates above and below the threshold for OCD at different periods.[11] In fact, there appears to be a large pool of subclinical OCD in the general population, estimated in one study to be as high as 19%.[12]

Although most children experience some obsessional symptoms during their development, in only a minority do the symptoms develop into OCD.[13] The lifetime prevalence in children has been reported to be almost as high as in adults, at around 2% (see Chapter 12). Of interest is the large proportion with obsessions only, exceeding 50% of the OCD respondents in one of the studies.

Age of onset

Retrospective studies suggest that the mean age of onset of OCD is earlier than that of depression, at around 20 years, with the incidence peaking once in the early teens and again in the early twenties. Males develop the disorder earlier than females (Figure 1.1).[14] Studies looking at children and adolescents with OCD reveal a similar pattern, with boys showing a prepubertal onset at around 9 years and girls developing the disorder around puberty.[15]

OCD and gender

Obsessive compulsive disorder is more common in women, although the differences are not as obvious as in depression or other anxiety disorders. An average female to male ratio of 1.5 : 1.0 is accepted for the community at large, although the ratio appears roughly equal in the adolescent population, reflecting perhaps the earlier onset in boys. In contrast, men predominate in surveys of OCD referrals, possibly reflecting a greater severity in males.

Women during pregnancy and the puerperium are particularly at risk of developing the disorder. In a study by Neziroglu et al of 59 mothers with OCD, 23 experienced their symptoms for the first time during pregnancy.[16] In many cases, pre-existing obsessional tendencies are unmasked and exaggerated by the events surrounding childbirth.

Familial factors

Obsessive compulsive disorder is considered to be one of the most strongly inherited mental disorders (see Chapter 6).[17] Approximately one-fifth of nuclear family members of OCD sufferers show signs of OCD, and the younger the sufferer the more likely they are to have a first-degree relative affected. The clustering of OCD and Tourette's syndrome (TS) within families suggests a common inherited factor.

Course and prognosis

The course of the illness can vary from a relatively benign form in which the patient experiences infrequent, discrete episodes of illness interspersed with symptom-free periods, to malignant OCD, characterized by unremitting symptoms and substantial social impairment.

In a 40-year prospective follow-up study, reported by Skoog and Skoog, the authors managed to locate and examine 144 out of 251 OCD patients who had previously been admitted as inpatients under their care between 1947 and 1953.[18] Given that effective treatments for OCD were not developed until the end of the study, much of the data is naturalistic. The authors found that roughly 60% showed signs of general improvement within 10 years of onset of illness, rising to 80% by the end of the study. However, only 20% achieved full remission even after nearly 50 years of illness; 60% continued to experience significant symptoms; 10% showed no improvement whatsoever; and another 10% had worsened. In 60% of cases the content of the obsessions shifted markedly over the follow-up period. One-fifth of those who had shown an early, sustained improvement subsequently relapsed, even after 20 years without symptoms, suggesting early recovery does not rule out the possibility of very late relapse. Intermittent, episodic disease was common during the early stage of illness, and predicted a more favourable outcome, whereas chronic illness predominated in the later years. Early age of onset, particularly in males, having both obsessions and compulsions or magical thinking, poor social adjustment, and an early chronic course, predicted a worse outcome.

A more recent 5-year prospective follow-up study of 100 OCD patients showed that in spite of the introduction of modern treatments, outcomes were similar to Skoog and Skoog's cohort, with only 20% reaching full remission of their OCD, 50% showing partial remission, and the remainder unchanged or worse over 5 years. Less severe illness and being married were associated with a better outcome.[19]

Symptoms and subtypes

Most patients suffer a mixture of different obsessions or compulsions. Surveys have consistently identified contamination fears as the most common obsession, with concern about harm to others, pathological doubt, somatic obsessions and the need for symmetry also occurring frequently. Half of all OCD patients admitted for treatment suffer compulsions in the realm of repetitive checking or excessive cleaning and washing (Table 1.3).[20] Key themes have been identified that underlie most symptoms. These include abnormal risk assessment, pathological doubt and incompleteness.[3]

Patients with OCD usually retain full insight into the absurdity of their symptoms, although this is not always the case.[21] The DSM-IV singles out patients with poor insight as a meaningful subgroup. These individuals have more complex symptomatology, which makes diagnosis more difficult, and tend to be more severely ill. They have only a limited sense of the excessiveness and irrationality of their thoughts and behaviours and are therefore difficult to engage in treatment. They may appear to be deluded (and hence receive inappropriate treatment) but longitudinal studies show they do not go on to develop schizophrenia-like illnesses.[22] In a cohort of 475 patients with OCD, 27 (6%) displayed lack of insight.[23]

Differential diagnosis

Mild forms of obsessional behaviour, such as repetitive checking or superstitious behaviour, commonly occur in everyday life. They only meet the criteria for OCD if they are time-consuming, or associated with impairment or distress.

Recurrent, intrusive thoughts, impulses and images also occur in other mental disorders thought to share a relationship with OCD: for example, the preoccupation with bodily appearance, in body dysmorphic disorder; with a feared object, in specific phobia; with illness, in hypochondriasis; or with hair-pulling, in trichotillomania. A diagnosis of OCD should only be

Table 1.3 Phenomenological analysis of 250 OCD inpatients.

Common obsessions (%)	Common compulsions (%)	
	Behaviours	Mental acts
Contamination fears (45%)	Checking (63%)	Covert counting (36%)
Repetitive doubts (42%)	Washing (50%)	
Somatic obsessions (36%)	Need to confess (36%)	
Need for symmetry (31%)	Ordering/symmetry (31%)	
Aggressive impulses (28%)	Hoarding (18%)	
Repeated sexual imagery (26%)		
Multiple obsessions (60%)	Multiple compulsions (48%)	

Adapted from Rasmussen and Eisen.[20]

made if there are also unrelated obsessive-compulsive symptoms, in which case more than one diagnosis may be warranted.

Activities such as preoccupation with eating, sex, shopping and gambling are not considered genuine compulsions because they are not egodystonic, and the individual usually only tries to resist because of the adverse consequences.

Comorbidity

Depression

Obsessive compulsive disorder shares comorbidity with a range of DSM Axis I and II disorders (Table 1.4), the most common of which is major depression. A diagnosis of OCD can be made in the presence of comorbid depression as long as the ruminations are not restricted to depressive themes. The ECA studies revealed that a third of adult patients with OCD also met the diagnostic criteria for major depression at the time of interview, and that three-quarters had suffered a major depressive episode at some point during the course of their OCD. Moreover, 12% of patients with a diagnosis of major depression also shared a lifetime diagnosis of OCD. In a large cohort study of children and adolescents with OCD, a third had a history of current or lifetime depression. The depression was equally likely to predate or follow the OCD.[24]

Studies have also shown higher rates of suicidal behaviour compared with patients suffering from other mental disorders. The suicidal behaviour appeared to be independent of concurrent depression.[25]

Many patients only present to doctors for treatment of their comorbid depression. In these cases it is important that the OCD is not missed, because the depression will only respond if the OCD is treated as well.[26]

Table 1.4   Comorbidity in OCD.

Diagnosis	Current (%)	Lifetime (%)
Major depression	31	67
Specific phobia	7	22
Social phobia	11	18
Eating disorder	8	17
Alcohol abuse	8	14
Panic disorder	6	12
Tourette's syndrome	5	17

Adapted from Rasmussen and Eisen.[20]

Tourette's syndrome

Tourette's syndrome (TS) is often complicated by comorbid OCD, with estimates ranging from 35% to 50%. The incidence of TS in OCD is lower (5–7%), although tics are reported in 20–30% of individuals with OCD. It has been postulated that some forms of OCD may represent a 'forme fruste' of TS. 'Uncomplicated' OCD patients have been reported to experience more contamination fears and cleaning and washing rituals, compared with obsessional patients with comorbid TS who reported more obsessive compulsive symptoms overall, and suffered more from aggressive, religious and sexual obsessions, forced touching, checking, counting and evening-up rituals.[27,28] Factor analysis of a large cohort of OCD sufferers identified four separate symptom clusters (obsessions and checking, symmetry and ordering, cleanliness and washing, and hoarding obsessions and compulsions) each with a different degree of heritability, suggesting the existence of biologically distinct subtypes.[29] This model needs to be reconciled with the finding that in most patients, changes occur in the content of the symptoms during the natural course of the illness.[18]

Obsessive compulsive personality disorder

The essential feature of obsessive compulsive personality disorder (OCPD) is a pervasive preoccupation with orderliness, perfectionism and mental and interpersonal control, at the expense of flexibility, openness and efficiency, which develops by early adulthood and persists (Table 1.5).[2] Unlike OCD, these traits are egosyntonic, and unacceptable obsessions and compulsions are absent.

According to psychoanalytical theory, OCD and OCPD share the same unconscious defence mechanisms, and OCD is thought to evolve out of OCPD. However, epidemiological studies consistently show that whereas

Table 1.5 Diagnostic specifiers for DSM-IV 301.4: obsessive compulsive personality disorder.

Preoccupation with details, rules, lists, order, organization or schedules
Perfectionism that interferes with task completion
Excessive devotion to work to the exclusion of leisure
Overconscientiousness, scrupulosity and inflexibility
Inability to discard worthless objects
Reluctance to delegate, needing to be in control
Miserliness
Rigidity and stubbornness

Adapted from DSM-IV.[2]

OCD sufferers are more likely than comparison subjects to have a personality disorder, OCPD is present in only a minority of cases, and is less common than mixed, dependent, avoidant and histrionic personality disorders. For example, in a study of 96 consecutive DSM-III OCD patients, only 6% fulfilled DSM criteria for OCPD using a standardized diagnostic instrument.[30] These findings indicate that OCPD is not a prerequisite for the development of OCD. In some cases OCD predates the development of personality disorders such as OCPD, and some experts have hypothesized that OCPD may develop as an adaptive response to long-standing OCD of early onset.

Schizophrenia

Distressing obsessions and compulsions affect 10–25% of schizophrenic patients, and these are often the most severely disabled and challenging cases. Preliminary findings suggest that the OCD requires separate treatment, since antipsychotic drugs are generally ineffective on their own and may occasionally make the OCD worse.[31]

Schizotypal personality disorder (SPD) is thought to be related to schizophrenia. It occurs in at least 5% of the OCD population, and is more common in the severely disabled group. Comorbid SPD confers a poor treatment outcome, and may be a common factor linking the other psychosocial indicators of poor prognosis including inadequate social function, poor treatment compliance, and poor insight.[30]

Somatic manifestations of OCD

One of the most common physical manifestations is dermatitis from excessive cleaning rituals. A screening of 92 patients attending a dermatology clinic by means of the Mini-International Neuropsychiatric Interview[22] revealed that approximately 20% scored positive either for OCD or for a clinically relevant spectrum disorder such as body dysmorphic disorder. In most cases the obsessional symptoms had not been previously diagnosed. Patients suffered from a variety of dermatological problems, most notably eczema and acne.

The genitourinary clinic is another area frequented by OCD sufferers with obsessions concerning sexually transmitted disease, nowadays mainly human immunodeficiency virus (HIV) infection. Patients with hypochondriacal obsessions present widely to hospital services, seeking medical reassurance, and their OCD usually escapes notice (Table 1.6). There is a need for a greater awareness of OCD in non-psychiatric health-care settings.

Table 1.6 Non-psychiatric health specialists likely to see patients with OCD.

Specialist	Presenting condition
Dermatologist	Chapped hands, eczema, trichotillomania, body dysmorphic disorder
General practitioner	Hypochondriasis
Oncologist	Fear of cancer
Genitourinary specialist	Fear of HIV
Neurologist	OCD associated with Tourette's syndrome
Obstetrician	OCD during pregnancy or the puerperium
Gynaecologist	Vaginal discomfort from douching

Raising the profile of OCD

Obsessive compulsive disorder is a secretive condition. Most patients are ashamed and confused by their illness. Many fear they are mad and actively disguise their symptoms to prevent discovery, and it usually takes years before they find a health professional in whom they feel they can confide (see Chapter 14). Untreated OCD is responsible for considerable social impairment and emotional morbidity.

Early recognition and accurate diagnosis are thus important public health objectives.[8] In spite of recent media publicity, lack of education remains a major problem. Although surveys suggest the time lag between onset of symptoms and correct diagnosis is shortening,[32] patients still wait on average 17 years before appropriate treatment is initiated.[8] Many practitioners are still unfamiliar with OCD and are unable to recognize or treat it correctly.

Increased awareness is the key to better recognition and treatment of OCD. Practitioners in areas known to attract high numbers of OCD sufferers should be primed to look for symptoms, and active screening for OCD using direct enquiry (e.g. Table 1.7) should be routinely incorporated into every mental state examination.

Table 1.7   Five questions to identify an OCD sufferer.

Do you wash or clean a lot?
Do you check things a lot?
Is there any thought that keeps bothering you that you would like to get rid of but can't?
Do your daily activities take a long time to finish?
Are you concerned about orderliness or symmetry?

Reproduced with kind permission of the International Council on OCD. Adapted from International Council on OCD, *Update on OCD* (Medical Action Communications: Egham, Surrey, UK 1995).

References

1 World Health Organization, *ICD 10 Classification of Mental and Behavioural Disorders. Clinical Descriptions and Diagnostic Guidelines* (WHO: Geneva, 1992).

2 American Psychiatric Association, *Diagnostic and Statistical Manual of Mental Disorders*, 4th edn (American Psychiatric Association: Washington, DC, 1994).

3 Rasmussen SA, Eisen JL, The epidemiology and differential diagnosis of obsessive compulsive disorder, *J Clin Psychiatry* (1992) **53**(suppl.):4–10.

4 Hollander E, Benzaquen SD, The obsessive-compulsive spectrum disorders, *Int Rev Psychiatry* (1997) **9**:99–109.

5 Robins LN, Holzer JE, Weissman MM et al, Lifetime prevalence of specific psychiatric disorders in three sites, *Arch Gen Psychiatry* (1984) **41**:949–58.

6 Myers J, Weissman M, Tischler G et al, Six month prevalence of psychiatric disorders in three communities, *Arch Gen Psychiatry* (1984) **41**:959–67.

7 Weissman MM, Bland RC, Canino GL et al, The cross national epidemiology of obsessive-compulsive disorder, *J Clin Psychiatry* (1994) **55**:5–10.

8 Hollander E, Wong C, Psychosocial functions and economic costs of obsessive compulsive disorder, *CNS Spectrums* (1998) **3**(5)suppl. 1:48–58.

9 Nelson E, Rice J, Stability of diagnosis of obsessive-compulsive disorder in the Epidemiological Catchment Area Study. *Am J Psychiatry* (1997) **154**:826–31.

10 Stein MB, Forde DR, Anderson G et al, Obsessive-compulsive disorder in the community: an epidemiological study with clinical reappraisal, *Am J Psychiatry* (1997) **154**:1120–6.

11 Degonda M, Wyss M, Angst J, The Zurich Study. XVIII. Obsessive compulsive disorders and syndromes in the general population, *Eur Arch Psychiat Clin Neurosci* (1993) **243**:16–22.

12 Valleni-Basile LA, Garrison CZ, Jackson KL et al, Frequency of obsessive compulsive disorder in a community sample of young adolescents, *J Am Acad Child Adolesc Psych* (1994) **33**:782–91.

13 Riddle MA, Scahill L, King R et al, Obsessive compulsive disorder in children and adolescents. *J Am Acad Child Adolesc Psych* (1990) **29**:766–72.

14 Rasmussen SA, Eisen JL. Epidemiology of obsessive compulsive disorder. *J Clin Psychiatry* (1990) **51**(suppl.):10–13.

15 Swedo SE, Rapoport JL, Leonard H et al, Obsessive compulsive disorder in children and adolescents: clinical phenomenology of 70 consecutive cases, *Arch Gen Psychiatry* (1989) **46**:335–41.

16 Neziroglu F, Anemone R, Yaryura-Tobias JA, Onset of obsessive compulsive disorder in pregnancy. *Am J Psychiatry* (1992) **149**:947–50.

17 Pauls DL, Alsobrook JP, Goodman W et al, A family study of obsessive compulsive disorder, *Am J Psychiatry* (1995) **152**:76–84.

18 Skoog G, Skoog I, A 40-year follow-up of patients with obsessive-compulsive disorder, *Arch Gen Psychiatry* (1999) **56**:121–7.

19 Steketee G, Eisen J, Dyck I et al, Predictors of course in obsessive compulsive disorder, *Psychiatr Res* (1999) **89**(3):229–38.

20 Rasmussen SA, Eisen JL, Epidemiology and clinical features of obsessive compulsive disorder. In: Jenike M, Baer L, Minichiello WE, eds, *Obsessive Compulsive Disorders. Theory and Management* (Year Book: Chicago, 1990) 10–27.

21 Insel T, Akiskal H, Obsessive compulsive disorder with psychotic features: a phenomenological analysis, *Am J Psychiatry* (1986) **143**:1527–33.

22 Sheehan DV, Lecrubier Y, Janavs J et al, Mini-international neuropsychiatric interview (MINI). University of South Florida Institute for Research in Psychiatry, Tampa, Fl, USA, and INSERM-Hôpital de la Salpetrière, Paris, France, 1994.

23 Eisen JL, Rasmussen SA, Obsessive compulsive disorder with psychotic features, *J Clin Psychiatry* (1993) **54**(10):373–9.

24 Swedo S, Rapoport S, Leonard H et al, Obsessive disorder in children and adolescents. *Arch Gen Psychiatry* (1989) **46**:335–41.

25 Hollander E, Greenwald S, Neville D et al, Uncomplicated and comorbid obsessive compulsive disorder in an epidemiological sample, *CNS Spectrums* (1998) **3**:(5)suppl. 1; 10–18.

26 Fineberg N, Evidence-based pharmacotherapy for obsessive-compulsive disorder, *Adv Psych Treatm* (1999) **5**:357–65.

27 Leckman JF, Grice DE, Barr LC et al, Tic-related vs. non-tic-related obsessive compulsive disorder, *Anxiety* (1994–5) **1**(5):208–15.

28 Eapen V, Robertson MM, Alsobrook JP et al, Obsessive compulsive symptoms in Gilles de la Tourette syndrome and obsessive compulsive disorder: differences by diagnosis and family history, *Am J Med Genet* (1997) **74**(4): 432–8.

29 Alsobrook JP, Leckman JF, Goodman WK et al, Segregation analysis of obsessive compulsive disorder using symptom-based factor scores, *Am J Med Genet* (1999) **88**(6):669–75.

30 Baer L, Jenike MA, Personality disorders in obsessive compulsive disorder, *Psychiatr Clin North Am* (1992) **15**(4):803–12.

31 Zohar J, Sasson Y, Chopra M et al, Schizo-obsessive subtype: obsessions and delusions, *CNS Spectrums* (1998) **3**(5)suppl. 1: 38–9.

32 Mallery E, The subjective experience of OCD. A questionnaire based study from members of the self-help organisation 'Obsessive Action'. Unpublished oral presentation to the Second Annual Conference of Obsessive Action, October 1996, Conway Hall, London.

2
Assessment of OCD

Toby D Goldsmith, Nathan A Shapira and Wayne K Goodman

As in the treatment of other illnesses, the appropriate diagnosis and assessment of obsessive compulsive disorder is imperative for proper management. Obsessive compulsive disorder (OCD) is a common psychiatric illness with a lifetime prevalence of 2.5% in the general population.[1] Because of embarrassment, patients are often reticent to present for treatment or spontaneously share their OCD symptoms with their caregiver.

The clinician must first determine if the diagnosis is appropriate. A thorough diagnostic evaluation is most effective. In addition to a clinical interview, the clinician may choose to have the patient complete either a screening tool to help validate the diagnostic evaluation or a rating scale to evaluate the extent of the symptoms. This information would be used to establish a baseline level of impairment. This chapter reviews the various tools that psychiatrists and other mental health professionals may use in the assessment of their patients.

Diagnostic tools

While face-to-face interviews are necessary for establishing rapport between patient and practitioner, a differential diagnosis may be initiated from information gathered during the interview. More structured screening tools not only further define diagnosis, but may determine the presence of additional psychiatric disorders from which the patient may suffer. There are both patient-administered and clinician-administered diagnostic and screening instruments; it is the clinician's choice which format is most useful in the given clinical setting.

The diagnosis of OCD symptoms can be confusing. Symptoms that appear to be obsessions may actually represent those of another disease (for example, ruminations in major depression or worries in generalized anxiety disorder). Tic disorders may be misdiagnosed as compulsions when the tics are complex, such as repetitive grooming and evening-up.

With appropriate training the clinician can learn to make distinctions between obsessions and compulsions and the other symptoms from which patients suffer.

Structured Clinical Interview for DSM-IV

The Structured Clinical Interview for DSM-IV (SCID-IV) is among the most widely used clinician-administered screening tools for OCD.[2] Its extensive categorized questions are useful when a complete differential diagnosis of Axis I disorders is desired. While completing the SCID-IV is time-consuming (especially in the presence of multiple diagnoses) the questions for each diagnosis are succinct, thus allowing for a quick determination if a particular diagnosis is present.

In university settings, the SCID-IV is generally carried out by a mental health clinician, such as a licensed psychologist, psychiatrist or social worker. For accurate diagnosis, the clinician must have appropriate training in using the SCID-IV. Between appropriately trained individuals, interrater reliability for the diagnosis of OCD is high, with a kappa score of 0.59 for a current diagnosis and 0.67 for a lifetime diagnosis.[3]

Anxiety Disorders Interview Schedule for DSM-IV

The Anxiety Disorders Interview Schedule for DSM-IV (ADIS-IV) is useful for establishing the presence or absence of psychiatric disorders.[4] The ADIS-IV is anxiety disorder-specific, unlike the SCID-IV; it also evaluates for highly comorbid diagnoses, such as affective disorders and substance abuse. For the clinician who requires a thorough assessment for anxiety disorders, the ADIS-IV is a more appropriate screening instrument than the SCID-IV.[5]

In the hands of a trained rater, the ADIS-IV may be a more reliable tool for diagnosing OCD than the SCID-IV, with an interrater reliability kappa score of 0.75 to 0.80.[6] Studies using the SCID-IV were performed differently from those using the ADIS-IV (multisite versus single site), which may account for the difference in kappa scores.

Rating instruments

Once the diagnosis of OCD is established, the clinician should determine the extent and severity of the symptoms. When symptoms are less severe, treatment may proceed at a more deliberate pace. In the presence of more significant symptoms and greater disability, the clinician may wish to approach treatment more aggressively. In addition, the results of rating tools may be useful in establishing a baseline for the patient's symptoms; repeated assessments after treatment has been initiated may be useful in tracking improvement and other changes, thus allowing for treatment adjustments. The diagnosis of OCD symptoms may be difficult. Some symptoms may be apparent only in specific environments, for example at home or at work. Because of embarrassment and shame, the patient may confound accurate assessment by concealing the degree of suffering. Patients may be reticent to share the exact nature of their obsessions and compulsions. Providing a supportive setting and ensuring confidentiality will assist in obtaining an accurate picture of the illness. With appropriate training a clinician can learn to derive an accurate view of the nature and severity of obsessions and compulsions.

Yale–Brown Obsessive Compulsive Scale

Although developed as a measurement tool for symptom severity and improvement in clinical drug trials, the Yale–Brown Obsessive Compulsive Scale (Y–BOCS, see Appendix 1, p. 183) has become the most widely used tool for assessing symptom severity.[7-9] It has been translated into more than a dozen languages. Unlike other measurement tools, the number of symptoms does not affect the Y–BOCS score; rather it assesses the extent to which the symptoms affect the individual's life.

The Y–BOCS consists of three sections. In the first, the clinician reads out to the patient descriptions and examples of obsessions and compulsions. Section two contains a symptom checklist of obsessions and compulsions; current and previous symptoms are identified during this section. The third consists of 10 core items and 11 investigational questions. The core items are rated by the clinician with a five-point scale (possible scores of 0–4), assessing the extent of symptoms. It is necessary that obsessions and compulsions are differentiated from the ruminations and ideations of other illnesses. The first item for both obsessions and compulsions defines the amount of time the patient spends on them, from 'no time' to 'more than 8 hours a day'. Other items review the patient's disruption and distress caused by the symptoms, and the resistance and control that are possible over these symptoms.[7] There are separate subtotal scores for both the obsession and compulsion sections. This allows a quantification of the illness when only one or the other symptom is present. This is allowable in the DSM-IV criteria for OCD.[10]

The investigational items for the Y–BOCS evaluate separately avoidance, indecisiveness, insight, pathological responsibility, slowness and doubting. Two additional questions are based on another inventory, the Clinical Global Impressions Scale.[11] A final item assesses the clinician's assessment of the reliability of the patient's report of symptoms. Investigational items are not added to the final Y–BOCS score of the core items.

When administering the Y–BOCS, it may be necessary to define obsessions and compulsions in terms of the patient's knowledge and understanding. During the second part of the evaluation, the patient is asked to specify both current and past obsessions and compulsions. These are based on the Y–BOCS symptom checklist; previous symptoms may resurface during treatment. Patient and clinician then describe the particular symptoms on the Y–BOCS target symptom list; those that are the most disturbing to the patient should be defined. Avoidance of certain situations is also recorded, since some patients limit their anxiety by shunning circumstances that evoke negative thoughts or feelings. Finally, the patient is asked to respond to the 19 core and investigational items; there may be circumstances when collateral information may be required to appropriately assess symptom severity (as in the case of children, or patients with little insight).

The Y–BOCS has been well studied and found to be a reliable instrument for determining symptom severity. Researchers have found it to have excellent interrater reliability and admirable test–retest reliability.[12–14] The Y–BOCS has also been found to be a good assessment tool for monitoring change in symptoms.[15–17] Changes in symptoms monitored by the Y–BOCS were specific for OCD and not for other anxiety disorders or depression.[8] Given the extent of validating research, clinicians can confidently use the Y–BOCS to assess the scope of their patients' illness.

The Y–BOCS has been modified into patient-administered screening tools. A computerized version may be used either in an office setting or administered by telephone.[18,19] Studies using both of these versions have found the tests to be consistent with clinician-administered versions of the Y–BOCS; normal control subjects, however, were noted to rate their symptoms as more significant than the trained raters, so this tool may not be appropriate for large-scale screening. However, it could be appropriately used for follow-up after a clinician-rated Y–BOCS has been administered. Two pen-and-paper forms have been developed as well, the Screening Test for Obsessive-compulsive Problems (STOP) for community-based settings and the Florida Obsessive Compulsive Inventory (FOCI) for clinics. Both consist of two parts determining the presence of symptoms, and the severity of these symptoms. The FOCI has more questions than the STOP and thus takes more time to administer. Little controlled data are available on either of these tests.

Maudsley Obsessional Compulsive Inventory

A 30-item true–false test, the Maudsley Obsessional Compulsive Inventory (MOCI, see Appendix 1, p. 216) was developed as a research tool to elucidate symptoms in previously diagnosed OCD patients.[20] The MOCI was derived from a larger set of items; this subset of the questions was determined to differentiate between patients with OCD and non-psychotic patients without OCD. There are four principal groups of OCD symptoms assessed by the MOCI: 'checking', 'cleaning', 'slowness', and 'doubting'. Each group can be scored individually. Unfortunately, OCD symptoms such as hoarding and aggression obsessions are not well examined by the MOCI. Given that the severity of symptoms is not scored, patients who have several symptoms will score higher than those with one or two symptoms even if both are equally disabled by the disorder. The MOCI has been found to be reliable and valid,[20] and in clinical drug trials it has been shown to detect symptom improvement, with small but significant changes from the baseline MOCI score.[21,22] This test is brief and easy to administer; however, it is limited in its scope of OCD symptoms and may not detect changes or improvement in symptoms.

Leyton Obsessional Inventory

The Leyton Obsessional Inventory (LOI) was used extensively prior to the introduction of the Y–BOCS.[23,24] This 69-question test can be used to assess obsessionality. For the clinician, the pen-and-paper version is the less cumbersome to administer. The LOI evaluates obsessional thoughts, although thoughts that are of a violent or other unacceptable nature are evaluated in less detail. The thoughts are scored in a dichotomous way. The level of resistance and interference with other activities are evaluated on a scale of 0–3 to help differentiate patients from those without OCD. An increased level of subjective disturbance is associated with a higher score. There are questions about the validity of the LOI.[25,26] It has not been found to be a consistent instrument for evaluating change in symptoms compared with other tools,[27,28] and thus the LOI may be less useful to the clinician in practice.

Padua Inventory

The Padua Inventory (PI), developed in 1988, was designed to improve the measurement of obsessive compulsive symptoms.[29] Its validity and reliability were tested on healthy volunteers and therefore its use in OCD is questionable. The revised version (PI-R), a 41-item tool, has been evaluated in OCD patients.[30] The 41 questions of the PI-R are divided into five sections: 'impulses', 'washing', 'checking', 'rumination' and 'precision'. This tool has been found to be reliable and consistent. The weakness of the PI-R lies in its inability to differentiate between obsessions and worries.[31] Further modifications of the PI have rectified this problem to an extent,[32] yet it may not completely differentiate OCD from depression or other anxiety disorders.

Conclusion

For the fastidious clinician, a diagnostic interview may only be the beginning of the evaluation process for OCD. A variety of assessment tools are used by researchers to elucidate the diagnosis and clarify the effects of treatment, and for the most part the statistical reliability and validity of these tools have been well established. Others may not be as sensitive or specific to the diagnosis of OCD, leading to the confusion of obsessions and compulsions with different psychiatric symptoms. For the clinician who wishes to administer testing for OCD, training in the administration and interpretation of these tools is essential. Well-educated clinicians may be pleased with the impact such training will have on their practice and their patients.

References

1 Robins LN, Helzer JE, Weissman MM et al, Lifetime prevalence of specific psychiatric disorders in three sites, *Arch Gen Psychiatry* (1984) **41**:949–58.

2 First MB, Spitzer RL, Gibbon M, Williams JBW, *Structured Clinical Interview for DSM-IV Axis I Disorders* – Patient edition (SCID-I/P, Version 2.0) (Biometrics Research Department, New York Psychiatric Institute: New York, 1996).

3 Williams JB, Gibbon M, First MB et al, The Structured Clinical Interview for DSM-III-R (SCID): II. Multisite test-retest reliability, *Arch Gen Psychiatry* (1992) **49**:630–6.

4 DiNardo P, Brown K, Barlow DH, *Anxiety Disorders Interview Schedule for DSM-IV* (Psychological Corporation: San Antonio, 1994).

5 Taylor S, Assessment of obsessive compulsive disorder. In: Swinson RP, Antony WM, Rachman S, Richter MA, eds, *Obsessive Compulsive Disorder: Theory, Research and Treatment* (Guilford Press: New York, 1998) 229–57.

6 DiNardo P, Moras K, Barlow DH, Rapee RM, Brown TA, Reliability of DSM-III-R anxiety disorders categories: using the Anxiety Disorders Interview Schedule-Revised (ADIS-R), *Arch Gen Psychiatry* (1993) **50**:251–6.

7 Goodman WK, Price LH, Rasmussen SA et al, The Yale–Brown Obsessive-Compulsive Scale. I. Development, use and reliability, *Arch Gen Psychiatry* (1989) **46**(11):1006–11.

8 Goodman WK, Price LH, Rasmussen SA et al, The Yale–Brown Obsessive-Compulsive Scale. II. Validity, *Arch Gen Psychiatry* (1989) **46**(11):1012–16.

9 Goodman WK, Rasmussen SA, Price LH, Mazure C, Heninger GR, Charney DS, *Manual for the Yale–Brown Obsessive Scale* (revised) (Connecticut Mental Health Center: New Haven, 1989).

10 American Psychiatric Association, *Diagnostic and Statistical Manual of Mental Disorders*, 4th edn (American Psychiatric Press: Washington, DC, 1994).

11 Guy W, *ECDEU Assessment Manual for Psychopharmacology*, publication no. 76-338 (US Department of Health, Education and Welfare: Washington, DC, 1976).

12 Kim SW, Dysken MW, Katz R, The Yale–Brown Obsessive-Compulsive Scale: a reliability and validity study. *Psychiatr Res* (1990) **34**: 99–106.

13 Kim SW, Dysken MW, Kuskowski MA, Hoover KM, The Yale–Brown

obsessive compulsive scale (Y-BOCS) and the NIMH global obsessive-compulsive scale (NIMH-GOCS): a reliability and validity study, *Int J Meth Psychiatr Res* (1993) **3**:37–44.

14 Woody SR, Steketee G, Chambless DL, Reliability, and validity of the Yale–Brown Obsessive-Compulsive Scale. *Behav Res Ther* (1995) **33**:597–605.

15 Clomipramine Collaborative Study Group, Clomipramine in the treatment of patients with obsessive compulsive disorder, *Arch Gen Psychiatry* (1991) **48**:730–8.

16 Tollefson GD, Rampey AH, Potvin JH et al, A multicenter investigation of fixed-dose fluoxetine in the treatment of obsessive compulsive disorder, *Arch Gen Psychiatry* (1994) **51**(7):559–67.

17 Wheadon DE, Bushnell WD, Steiner M, A fixed dose comparison of 20, 40 or 60 mg Paroxetine to placebo in the treatment of obsessive compulsive disorder [abstract]. (ACNP: Hawaii, 1993).

18 Baer L, Brown-Beasely MW, Sorce J, Henriques A, Computer-assisted telephone administration of a structured interview for obsessive compulsive disorder, *Am J Psychiatry* (1993) **150**: 1737–8.

19 Rosenfeld R, Dar R, Anderson D, Koback KA, Greist JH, A computer-administered version of the Yale–Brown Obsessive-Compulsive Scale, *Psychol Assess* (1992) **4**:329–32.

20 Hodgson RJ, Rachman S, Obsessional-compulsive complaints, *Behav Res Ther* (1977) **15**:389–95.

21 Goodman WK, Price LH, Rasmussen SA, Delgado PL, Heninger GR, Charney DS, Efficacy of fluvoxamine in obsessive compulsive disorder. A double-blind comparison with placebo, *Arch Gen Psychiatry* (1989) **46**(1):36–44.

22 Perse TL, Greist JH, Jefferson JW, Rosenfeld R, Dar R, Fluvoxamine treatment of obsessive compulsive disorder, *Am J Psychiatry* (1987) **144**:1543–8.

23 Cooper J, The Leyton obsessional inventory, *Psychol Med* (1970) **1**(1):48–64.

24 Snowdon J, A comparison of written and postbox forms of the Leyton Obsessional Inventory, *Psychol Med* (1980) **10**:165–70.

25 Clark DA, Bolton D, An investigation of two self report measures of obsessional phenomena in obsessive-compulsive adolescents. Research note, *J Child Psychol Psychiatry* (1985) **26**:429–37.

26 Philpott R, Recent advances in the behavioural measurement of obsessional illness. Difficulties common to these and other instruments, *Scott Med J* (1975) **20**:33–40.

27 Insel TR, Murphy DL, Cohen RM, Alterman I, Kilts C, Linnoila M, Obsessive compulsive disorder: a double-blind trial of Clomipramine and clorgyline, *Arch Gen Psychiatry* (1983) **40**:605–12.

28 Thoren P, Asberg M, Cronholm B et al, Clomipramine treatment of obsessive compulsive disorder I: a controlled clinical trial, *Arch Gen Psychiatry* (1980) **37**:1281–5.

29 Sanavio E, Obsessions and compulsions: the Padua Inventory, *Behav Res Ther* (1988) **28**: 314–45.

30 Van Oppen P, Hoekstra RJ, Emmelkamp PMG, The structure of obsessive-compulsive symptoms, *Behav Res Ther* (1995) **33**: 15–23.

31 Freestone MH, Ladouceur R, Rheaume J, Letarte H, Gagnon F, Thibodeau N, Self-report of obsessions and worry, *Behav Res Ther* (1994) **32**:29–36.

32 Burns GL, Keortge SG, Formea GM, Sternberger LG, Revision of the Padua Inventory for obsessive compulsive disorder symptoms: distinctions between worry, obsessions and compulsions, *Behav Res Ther* (1996) **34**: 163–73.

3

Obsessive compulsive spectrum disorders: from serotonin to dopamine and back again

Michael Van Ameringen, Jonathan M Oakman, Catherine Mancini and Peter Farvolden

A variety of similarities have been observed among a number of psychiatric and neuropsychiatric conditions and obsessive compulsive disorder (OCD). Some researchers suggest that this wide range of disorders shares enough similar features with OCD to be meaningfully grouped with it. The set of candidate disorders includes: somatoform disorders such as somatization disorder, hypochondriasis and body dysmorphic disorder; eating disorders (anorexia nervosa, bulimia nervosa, binge eating disorder); impulse control disorders such as problem gambling, kleptomania, compulsive buying, and trichotillomania; the paraphilias and non-paraphilic sexual addictions; Axis II disorders such as borderline and obsessive compulsive personality disorder; onychophagia (severe nail-biting), psychogenic excoriation (compulsive skin-picking) and repetitive self-mutilation. The list may also include disorders such as Tourette's syndrome, autism and Asperger's syndrome, and neurological conditions such as Sydenham's chorea. This group of disorders has been collectively referred to as the obsessive compulsive (OC) spectrum of disorders.[1–3] One common feature of these conceptual schemes is that OCD is thought to be the prototype for this group of disorders.

While many researchers seem to share the opinion that OCD is the prototype disorder of the OC spectrum, the disorder itself defies prototypal characterization. The presentation of OCD is heterogeneous; there is little to suggest a set of common elements and at least some evidence to suggest that there may be several different prototypes. These diverse presentations may be clinically discrete, being based on different neuropsychological substrates and having different treatment responses. Furthermore, these different types of OCD may be co-transmitted with different putative spectrum disorders. Hollander and Wong suggest a subdivision of OCD into five subtypes:

1. an obsessive compulsive personality subtype
2. an obsessional slowness subtype

3. a poor insight subtype
4. a harm-avoidant, adult-onset, non-tic-related subtype
5. a symmetry, childhood-onset, 'just so', tic-related subtype.

An alternative system of three subtypes derives from the factor analytic work of Baer:[4]

1. 'symmetry/hoarding' (impulsions)
2. 'contamination/cleaning' (compulsions)
3. 'pure obsessions'.

To the extent that the subtypes proposed in either of these systems represent meaningful categories of OCD, it may be more appealing to think in terms of multiple spectra of OCD, rather than a single unified OCD spectrum.

Conceptualizations of the OCD spectrum

There are a number of different conceptualizations of the OC spectrum.[5–8] Jarry and Vaccarino proposed that OCD and eating disorders are connected by an approach/avoidance continuum.[6] The contamination concerns of OCD and the restricting behaviour of anorexia are characterized by excessive avoidance. The sexual and violent obsessions of OCD and the gorging of bulimia are characterized by excessive approach. Alternatively, Hollander and Rosen proposed a dimension of compulsivity and impulsivity to explain a subset of the OCD spectrum, with OCD and body dysmorphic disorder at the compulsive end, and borderline and antisocial personality disorders at the impulsive end.[5] Hollander and Rosen suggest that the compulsive end of the dimensions is characterized by harm overestimation, while the impulsive end is characterized by underestimation of harm. Similarly, McElroy, Phillips and Keck argue that the OCD spectrum disorders are unified by a common core of compulsivity and/or impulsivity.[7] They argue for broadening the OCD spectrum to include all conditions characterized by obsessional thinking or behavioural stereotypies. In contrast, Rasmussen cautions that such an inclusive scheme may be unwarranted; many of the putative OCD spectrum disorders may be unrelated to OCD, and OCD itself may be a heterogeneous set of illnesses.[8,9] Rasmussen argues that there may be three core features of OCD, including abnormal risk assessment, pathological doubt, and incompleteness, and that these core features connect with some of the OCD spectrum disorders. Abnormal risk assessment is often comorbid with other obsessional illnesses such as generalized anxiety disorder or social phobia, while incompleteness is often comorbid with tics or habit disorders such as trichotillomania.

There is better evidence for the grouping of some of the OCD spectrum disorders with OCD and with each other than for others. For example, Bienvenu et al conducted a family study of OCD and found that body dysmorphic disorder may be co-transmitted with OCD, while the evidence was considerably weaker for other disorders.[10] Similarly, the evidence concerning the association of obsessive compulsive personality disorder with OCD is very weak.[11–13] It is possible that in our zeal to group similar disorders we have been overinclusive. It stretches a point to argue that all disorders that involve repetitive behaviour, intrusive thoughts and behaviour that is experienced as 'compelled' are all somehow related to OCD. Some have argued that most psychopathological conditions and a great deal of normal behaviour involves some degree of stereotypy, if stereotypy is broadly construed.[2]

The tic-related subtype of OCD and related disorders

While much of the current theorizing about OC spectrum disorders is speculative, there is substantial evidence that suggests an important relationship between OCD and tic disorders, including Tourette's syndrome.[14] At present the clearest distinction to be made among *subtypes* of OCD is the distinction between tic-related and non-tic-related OCD. In this chapter we will focus on tic-related OCD and the disorders that may go with it. We group some spectrum disorders with tic-related OCD partly on the basis of phenomenology and comorbidity, but in doing so we propose a dimension that describes the relationship between OCD and some of the other potential OC spectrum disorders that goes beyond simple descriptive similarities and has implications for treatment.

Tourette's syndrome (TS) is characterized by motor tics and one or more vocal tics beginning before the age of 18 years.[15] The tics of TS can share some phenomenological similarities with the compulsions of OCD.[16,17] People with TS report that while they can delay their tics, they find them irresistible, experience relief when they perform them, and sometimes need to perform them until they are 'just right'.[17] People with TS also report experiencing sensory phenomena prior to or concomitant with their tics that can resemble OCD obsessions, and that their tics are exacerbated by stress.[16] Obsessive compulsive disorder and OCD symptoms are common in patients with TS, with observed rates ranging from 12% to 90%,[16,17] and patients with OCD have been found to have high rates (37–59%) of tics and tic disorders.[18,19]

The most striking similarity between TS and OCD is that both are characterized by repetitive behaviour that is apparently senseless. Considerable attention has recently been turned to the task of classifying repetitive behaviours or stereotypies in terms of subjective experience.[4,20,21] The compulsions typical of OCD are defined in DSM-IV as 'repetitive behaviors . . . or mental acts . . . the goal of which is to prevent or reduce anxiety or distress, not to provide pleasure or gratification'.[15] Somewhat unlike classic compulsions are 'impulsions', which are spontaneous actions usually precipitated by a sensation or an urge and which are performed until a sense of 'rightness' or satisfaction is achieved.[22] Impulsions are not intended to neutralize an event or obsession but rather are intended to achieve a sense of completion, relief or satisfaction. Finally, there are tics. Tics may be simple or complex, and may be experienced as completely involuntary spontaneous muscle twitches or spasms, or as unvoluntary – based on an urge or sensation that is relieved by the tic.

According to the conceptual scheme outlined above, some classic OCD symptoms are impulsions, and others are compulsions. Checking behaviour would be a compulsion, as it reduces the anxiety brought on by an obsessive thought. Symmetry, hoarding and repeating would be impulsions, as they are typically performed until a sense of rightness is achieved.

Miguel and his colleagues compared three groups of patients: a group with OCD without tics or TS, a group of TS patients without OCD, and a group of patients with both OCD and TS.[14,20] They found that for OCD patients without comorbid tics or TS, repetitive behaviour was preceded by cognitive phenomena (obsessive thoughts or images) and anxiety, but largely not by sensory phenomena. In contrast, the TS group and the group with OCD and comorbid TS reported more sensory phenomena and fewer cognitions than the OCD group. These results support earlier findings by George et al, who found that patients with both OCD and comorbid TS reported that their repetitive behaviour arose spontaneously, while patients with OCD alone reported cognitions preceding repetitive behaviour.[23] Furthermore, Rasmussen and Eisen noted that OCD patients with primary concerns about symmetry (an impulsion) reported a feeling of discontent or tension rather than the experience of anxiety.[24]

Obsessive compulsive disorder with comorbid tics also seems to respond differently to treatment compared with more compulsive OCD. Antidepressants that target serotonergic systems are effective in the treatment of OCD,[25–27] while neuroleptics alone are ineffective.[28] In contrast, TS does not respond to antiobsessional drugs such as clomipramine and fluoxetine, but does respond to neuroleptic medication.[22,29–31] Moreover, there is a growing body of research evidence suggesting that OCD with comorbid tics is less responsive to serotonin reuptake inhibiting (SRI) drugs alone, but does respond better to a combination of SRIs and neuroleptic medication.[32,33] Case studies and open trials (for example that of McDougle et al,[32] reviewed by Goodman et al[28] have been followed by a controlled investigation of neuroleptic augmentation of SRIs.[33] The results of these investigations persuaded McDougle et al, among others, to argue that OCD with comorbid tics is a clinically meaningful subtype of OCD.[33]

If we think of the phenomenology of impulsions and tics as being related to dopaminergic systems and the phenomenology of obsessions and compulsions as being more serotonergic, then other disorders that share this phenomenology may be characterized in this way. Putative spectrum disorders that have an obsessive phenomenology should be more related to classic obsessional OCD than to tic-related OCD, and should respond well to SRI treatment. Disorders that have a tic-like phenomenology, or for which the main symptoms are impulsions, should be more associated with tic-related OCD and dopamine antagonists may provide useful treatment augmentation. A prime example of a disorder that is described by sufferers as like an impulsion is trichotillomania.

Trichotillomania is categorized as an impulse control disorder in DSM-IV.[15] The cardinal symptoms of the disorder are pulling out one's hair, resulting in noticeable hair loss; an increasing subjective sense of tension immediately preceding pulling out the hair or when attempting to inhibit the desire; and a resulting feeling of relief, gratification or pleasure when pulling out the hair. Trichotillomania is often considered to be part of the OC spectrum.[34]

Considering the symptom-based subtyping of OCD proposed by Baer,[4] the hair-pulling behaviour in trichotillomania would be an impulsion, as hair-pulling is typically not preceded by an obsessive thought but by an urge to pull,[35] and is followed by tension relief.[36] Hair-pulling is an end in itself, and does not serve to reduce anxiety.[36] Phenomenologically, trichotillomania seems more like TS or 'impulsive' OCD than classic 'compulsive' OCD.

Published evidence is equivocal on the efficacy of fluoxetine and other SRIs in the treatment of trichotillomania (for a review see Yanchick et al).[37] Swedo and her colleagues conducted a double-blind, crossover comparison of the treatment of trichotillomania in children with clomipramine and desipramine, finding that clomipramine treatment resulted in greater symptom reduction and overall improvement than desipramine.[38] Despite these promising initial results, effective treatment of trichotillomania with SRIs has not replicated well.[39–41]

Treating trichotillomania with medications typically used in the treatment of OCD has been largely unsuccessful, or at least much less successful than the treatment of OCD with these medications. A number of researchers have reported promising results with augmentation of SRI agents with a variety of dopaminergic agents including pimozide (a dopamine antagonist),[35] risperidone,[40] and haloperidol.[42] Finally, Ninan et al reported significant therapeutic benefit in an open trial of venlafaxine in trichotillomania; they argued that the benefit observed was probably due to venlafaxine's powerful inhibition of norepinephrine (noradrenaline) as well as serotonin reuptake.[43] However, it is interesting to note that one of the secondary binding properties of venlafaxine is on dopamine reuptake.[44] In summary, there is now considerable evidence for a role for dopaminergic agents in the treatment of trichotillomania.

It may be useful to think of at least some OC spectrum disorders as falling on a continuum anchored by two poles, with classic 'compulsive' OCD at one end, and with TS and attendant tic behaviour at the other. Trichotillomania may be thought of as closer to TS than to OCD on this tentative axis. The continuum we propose is only one dimension, accounting for a small subset of the OCD spectrum disorders. Classic compulsive OCD may be relatively serotonergic, while tic-related OCD may have an additional dopaminergic influence and may go with trichotillomania, skin-picking, nail-biting and TS. Phenomenologically speaking, the dimension seems to range from compulsive behaviour to tics, with impulsions being in between (Figure 3.1). The implication for the treatment is that there is likely to be some promise for dopaminergic agents in the treatment of disorders such as trichotillomania, skin-picking and nail-biting.

Clearly, serotonergic systems are important in OCD and the OC spectrum disorders. A variety of evidence, apart from treatment response and the results of pharmacological challenge studies, supports an important role for serotonin (5-HT) systems in the pathogenesis of OC spectrum disorders. For example, serotonergic projections from raphe to limbic structures are involved in anxiety and panic.[44] However, current evidence suggests an important role for other neurotransmitters as well. The fact remains that only 50–60% of patients with OCD demonstrate a decrease in OCD symptoms after long-term treatment with an SRI.[2] While there may be evidence for a role for norepinephrine, opioid and hormonal systems in some of the OC spectrum disorders, the best evidence points to a centrally important role for dopamine in the OC spectrum.[33]

Dopamine and the OC spectrum

There are four well-defined dopamine pathways in the brain: the nigrostriatal, mesolimbic, mesocortical, and tuberoinfundibular pathways (Figure 3.2).[44] One way to move towards a better understanding of the OC spectrum disorders may be found in research that examines the functioning of these pathways across various disorders.

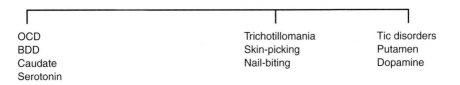

OCD   Trichotillomania   Tic disorders
BDD   Skin-picking   Putamen
Caudate   Nail-biting   Dopamine
Serotonin

Figure 3.1

Trichotillomania and the obsessive compulsive spectrum. BDD, body dysmorphic disorder; OCD, obsessive compulsive disorder.

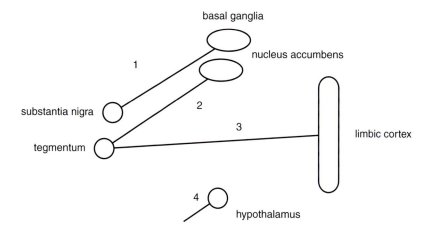

Figure 3.2

Dopamine pathways in the brain: 1, nigrostriatal; 2, mesolimbic; 3, mesocortical; 4, tuberoinfundibular.

The nigrostriatal dopamine pathway is a part of the extrapyramidal motor system and controls motor movements. This pathway projects from dopaminergic cell bodies in the substantia nigra of the brainstem via axons terminating in the basal ganglia.[44] The basal ganglia are composed of a set of intimately connected structures that include the caudate and putamen (striatum), globus pallidus, substantia nigra and subthalamic nucleus. Approximately 80% of all synapses in the striatum are cortical inputs. The cortical areas projecting to the striatum can be roughly divided into 'motor' areas, which include somatosensory, motor and premotor cortices, and 'limbic associative' areas, which include amygdala, hippocampus, and orbital, entorhinal, temporal, prefrontal, parietal, cingulate and association cortex. A similar level of division can be maintained at the level of the striatum, with a 'motor' putamen and a 'limbic' caudate and ventral striatum (nucleus accumbens).[45]

While Tourette's syndrome is most often associated with dysfunction of the putamen, OCD is most often associated with dysfunction of the caudate.[46] Indeed, it seems likely that involvement of the ventromedial caudate nucleus, receiving projections from the anterior orbitofrontal cortex, leads to the affectively tinged cognitive symptoms of OCD, whereas involvement of the putamen, receiving projections from sensorimotor cortices, leads to the somatosensory premonitory symptoms and tics of TS.[47] It is interesting to note that morphometric magnetic resonance imaging studies suggest that patients with trichotillomania exhibit subtle volumetric abnormalities of the putamen, as do patients with TS.[48] It may be that skin-picking and onychophagia (severe nail-biting) will also be found to be associated with relatively more dopaminergic (nigrostriatal) and putamen dysfunction.

The mesolimbic dopamine pathway projects from dopaminergic cell bodies in the ventral tegmental area of the brainstem to axon terminals in the limbic area of the brain, such as the nucleus accumbens. The nucleus accumbens is thought to be involved in many behaviours including pleasurable sensations, the powerful euphoria of drugs of abuse, as well as the delusions and hallucinations of psychosis.[44] Obsessive compulsive disorder with psychotic features or OC spectrum disorders that are characterized by delusional obsessions, as is sometimes observed in somatization disorder, hypochondriasis and the eating disorders,[49] may be associated with dysfunction of the mesolimbic system.

Stimulation of mesolimbic structures, especially the ventral tegmentum, leads to an immediate and sustained increase in extracellular dopamine in the nucleus accumbens. This increase in dopamine levels is thought to be the physiologic correlate of reward. Indeed, the mesolimbic dopamine pathway and nucleus accumbens appear to be the final common pathway for the positive reinforcement of a number of survival behaviours such as eating, drinking and copulation, as well as that of addictive drugs.[50]

Obsessive compulsive spectrum disorders including problem gambling,[51] compulsive buying, compulsive sexual behaviour, and perhaps bulimia nervosa, could be viewed as addictive disorders in which the mesolimbic dopamine pathway is dysfunctional. However, there is more to addictive behaviour than dopamine and the nucleus accumbens. There is considerable interest in the role of affect regulation in maintaining addictive behaviours and it seems likely that serotonergic and noradrenergic mechanisms play an important part in these processes.[52] In addition, serotonin and glutamate seem to share a role in the plasticity of sensitization and learning addictive behaviours, and norepinephrine seems to be related to risk-taking that crosses diagnostic boundaries.[50]

Cell bodies for the mesocortical dopamine pathway arise in the ventral tegmental area of the brainstem and project to various areas of the cerebral cortex, especially the limbic cortex. Some researchers believe that the negative and cognitive symptoms of schizophrenia are due to a deficit of dopamine to mesocortical projection areas, such as the dorsolateral prefrontal cortex.[44,53] Relatively non-specific symptoms that may or may not be present across the OC spectrum disorders and may be associated with mesolimbic dopamine pathway dysfunction include cognitive impairment, attentional problems, affective flattening, poverty of speech, psychomotor retardation and hoarding.[47,53,54]

Tuberoinfundibular pathway dopamine neurons project from the hypothalamus to the anterior pituitary.[44] Increased prolactin levels are associated with increased grooming and sexual behaviour.[55] Thus, OC spectrum disorders associated with tuberoinfundibular dopamine pathway may include trichotillomania, skin-picking, onychophagia, and perhaps compulsive sexual behaviour.

. . . and back to serotonin again

Rauch and Savage have proposed a model of the functional anatomy and organization of corticostriatal pathways in which they distinguish between sensorimotor, oculomotor, dorsal cognitive, ventral cognitive and affective-motivational corticostriatal circuits (Figure 3.3).[46] The sensorimotor circuit projects from primary and associated sensorimotor cortex via the putamen, to the ventral tier nuclei of the thalamus. The oculomotor circuit projects primarily from frontal eye fields via the body of the caudate nucleus, to the ventral anterior and medial dorsal nuclei of the thalamus, and plays a part in eye movements. The dorsal cognitive circuit projects primarily from the dorsal, anterior and lateral regions of the prefrontal cortex via the dorsolateral portion of the head of the caudate nucleus to the ventral anterior and medial dorsal nuclei of the thalamus. The dorsal cognitive circuit is thought to have a role in cognitive processes including working memory and the ability to establish and shift mental sets. The ventral cognitive circuit projects from the anterior and

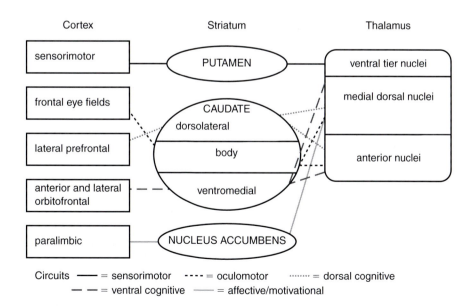

Figure 3.3

Functional anatomy and organization of corticostriatal pathways.

lateral orbitofrontal cortex via the ventromedial portion of the caudate nucleus, as well as to the ventral anterior and medial dorsal nuclei of the thalamus, and has an important role in cognitive processes such as response inhibition, especially as related to social or emotional subject matter. The affective-motivational circuit projects from paralimbic cortical territories (i.e. the posteromedial orbitofrontal cortex and the anterior cingulate) via the nucleus accumbens (i.e. the ventral striatum) to the medial dorsal nucleus within the thalamus. This circuit is also influenced heavily by limbic structures, such as the amygdala, and has a role in emotional or reward-based information processing.

An assumption that a model of functional anatomy and organization of corticostriatal pathways such as that proposed by Rauch and Savage is roughly accurate provides one reasonable way to further understand the relationship between such circuits and the OC spectrum disorders. For example, it may be that certain of the circuits (e.g. sensorimotor, oculomotor and affective-motivational circuits) are more vulnerable to dopaminergic dysfunction, while other circuits (e.g. dorsal and ventral cognitive circuits) are more dependent on serotonergic functioning.

Clearly, serotonergic dysfunction is important in the pathogenesis of OCD and many OC spectrum disorders. However, there is evidently more to OCD and OC spectrum disorders than serotonergic dysfunction alone. Symptoms of obsessions and compulsive washing, checking and cleaning are probably associated with functional changes in the caudate and orbitofrontal cortex as well as dysregulation of serotonergic functioning, and this is also likely to be true of OC spectrum disorders such as body dysmorphic disorder and perhaps hypochondriasis. In contrast, Tourette's syndrome is associated with functional changes in the putamen and dysregulation of dopaminergic functioning. 'Impulsive' OC spectrum disorders such as trichotillomania and perhaps skin-picking and onychophagia seem much more like TS than OCD. In this view patients with OCD and comorbid tics are likely to have functional changes in caudate, putamen and orbitofrontal cortex, and dysregulation in both serotonergic and dopaminergic systems.

One road towards a better understanding of the OC spectrum disorders may be found in research that examines the functioning of various serotoninergic, dopaminergic and noradrenergic pathways and the functional anatomy and organization of corticostriatal pathways across various disorders.[47] For example, it seems likely that dopamine (approach/reward), serotonin (learning, mood, impulsivity), norepinephrine (risk-taking) and the opiate system all have a role in the initiation and maintenance of addictive behaviours and perhaps some 'addiction-like' OC spectrum disorders including problem gambling, compulsive buying, compulsive sexual behaviour, and perhaps bulimia nervosa.

While the outline of a potential understanding of the variety of putative OC spectrum disorders presented here has been brief, we hope it encourages the interested clinician to think beyond the 'chicken bones' of patterns of comorbidity. Certainly the field needs more clinicians and researchers who are willing to move towards testable models of the OC spectrum based on consideration of ethology, neurobiology and treatment response.[2,47]

References

1　Hollander E, Wong CM, Spectrum, boundary, and subtyping issues: implications for treatment-refractory obsessive-compulsive disorder. In: Goodman WK, Rudorfer MV, Magser J, eds, *Obsessive-Compulsive Disorder: Contemporary Issues in Treatment* (Lawrence Erlbaum: Mahwah, 2000).

2　Stein DJ, Advances in the neurobiology of obsessive-compulsive disorder: implications for conceptualizing putative obsessive-compulsive and spectrum disorders, *Psychiatr Clin North Am* (2000) **23**(3):545–61.

3　Goldsmith T, Shapira NA, Phillips KA, McElroy SL, Conceptual foundations of obsessive-compulsive spectrum disorders. In: Swinson RP, Antony MM, Rachman S, Richter MA, eds, *Obsessive-Compulsive Disorder: Theory, Research and Treatment* (Guilford Press: New York, 1998).

4　Baer L, Factor analysis of symptom subtypes of obsessive-compulsive disorder and their relation to personality and tic disorders, *J Clin Psychiatry* (1994) **55**(3, suppl.):18–23.

5　Hollander E, Rosen J, Impulsivity, *J Psychopharmacol* (2000) **14**(2 suppl.):S39–44.

6　Jarry JL, Vaccarino FJ, Eating disorder and obsessive-compulsive disorder: neurochemical phenomenological commonalities, *J Psych Neurosci* (1996) **21**(1):36–48.

7　McElroy SL, Phillips KA, Keck PE, Obsessive compulsive spectrum disorder, *J Clin Psychiatry* (1994) **55**(suppl.):33–51.

8　Rasmussen SA, Obsessive compulsive spectrum disorders, *J Clin Psychiatry* (1994) **55**(3):89–91.

9　Rasmussen S, Eisen JL, The epidemiology and differential diagnosis of obsessive compulsive disorder, *J Clin Psychiatry* (1994) **55**(suppl.):5–10.

10　Bienvenu OJ, Samuels JF, Riddle MA et al, The relationship of obsessive-compulsive disorder to possible spectrum disorders: results from a family study, *Biol Psychiatry* (2000) **48**:287–93.

11　Rosen KV, Tallis F, Investigation into the relationship between personality traits and OCD, *Behav Res Ther* (1995) **33**(4):445–50.

12　Black DW, Noyes R, Pfohl B, Goldstein RB, Blum N, Personality disorders in OCD volunteers, well-comparison subjects, and their first degree relatives, *Am J Psychiatry* (1993) **150**(8):1226–32.

13　Thomsen PH, Mikkelssen HU, Development of personality disorders in children and adolescents in obsessive-compulsive disorder: a 6 to 22 year follow-up study, *Acta Psychiatr Scand* (1993) **87**(6):456–62.

14　Miguel EC, Coffey BJ, Baer L, Savage CR, Rauch SL, Jenike MA, Phenomenology of intentional repetitive behaviors in obsessive-compulsive disorder and Tourette's disorder, *J Clin Psychiatry* (1995) **56**:246–55.

15   American Psychiatric Association, *Diagnostic and Statistical Manual of Mental Disorders*, 4th edn (American Psychiatric Press: Washington, 1994).

16   Como PG, Obsessive-compulsive disorder in Tourette's syndrome, *Adv Neurol* (1995) **65**:281–91.

17   Leckman JF, Walker DE, Goodman WK, Pauls DL, Cohen DJ, 'Just right' perceptions associated with compulsive behavior in Tourette's syndrome, *Am J Psychiatry* (1994) **151**(5):675–80.

18   Leonard HL, Lenane MC, Swedo SE, Rettew DC, Gershon ES, Rapoport JL, Tics and Tourette's disorder: a 2- to 7-year follow-up of 54 obsessive-compulsive children, *Am J Psychiatry* (1992) **149**(9):1244–51.

19   Pitman RK, Green RC, Jenike MA, Mesulam MM, Clinical comparison of Tourette's disorder and obsessive-compulsive disorder, *Am J Psychiatry* (1987) **144**(9): 1166–71.

20   Miguel EC, Baer L, Coffey BJ et al, Phenomenological differences appearing with repetitive behaviours in obsessive-compulsive disorder and Gilles de la Tourette's syndrome, *Br J Psychiatry* (1997) **170**:104–45.

21   Tourette Syndrome Classification Study Group, Definitions and classification of tic disorders, *Arch Neurol* (1993) **50**:1013–16.

22   Shapiro AK, Shapiro E, Evaluation of the reported association of obsessive-compulsive symptoms or disorder with Tourette's disorder, *Compr Psychiatry* (1992) **33**:152–65.

23   George MS, Trimble MR, Ring HA, Sallee FR, Robertson MM, Obsessions in obsessive-compulsive disorder with and without Gilles de la Tourette's syndrome, *Am J Psychiatry* (1993) **150**(1):93–7.

24   Rasmussen S, Eisen JL, Phenomenology of OCD: clinical subtypes, heterogeneity and coexistence. In: Zohar J, Insel I, Rasmussen S, eds, *The Psychobiology of Obsessive-Compulsive Disorder* (Springer: New York, 1991) 13–43.

25   Jenike MA, Baer L, Summergrad P, Weilburg JB, Holland A, Seymour R, Obsessive-compulsive disorder: a double-blind, placebo-controlled trial of clomipramine in 27 patients, *Am J Psychiatry* (1989) **146**:1328–30.

26   Jenike MA, Hyman S, Baer L et al, A controlled trial of fluvoxamine in obsessive-compulsive disorder: implications for a serotonergic theory, *Am J Psychiatry* (1990) **147**:1209–15.

27   Goodman WK, Price LH, Rasmussen SA, Delgado PL, Heninger GR, Charney DS, Efficacy of fluvoxamine in obsessive-compulsive disorder: a double-blind comparison with placebo, *Arch Gen Psychiatry* (1989) **26**:123–8.

28   Goodman WK, McDougle CJ, Price LH, Riddle MA, Pauls DL, Leckman JF, Beyond the serotonin hypothesis: a role for dopamine in some forms of obsessive-compulsive disorder, *J Clin Psychiatry* (1990) **51**:36–43.

29   Shapiro AK, Shapiro E, Treatment of Gilles de la Tourette's syndrome with haloperidol, *Br J Psychiatry* (1968) **114**:345–50.

30   Shapiro AK, Shapiro ES, The treatment and etiology of tics and Tourette's syndrome, *Compr Psychiatry* (1981) **22**:193–205.

31   Shapiro AK, Shapiro E, Young JG, *Gilles de la Tourette Syndrome*, 2nd edn (Raven Press: New York, 1988).

32   McDougle CJ, Goodman WK, Price JH et al, Neuroleptic addition in fluvoxamine-refractory

obsessive-compulsive disorder, *Am J Psychiatry* (1990) **147**: 652–4.

33 McDougle CJ, Goodman WK, Leckman JF, Lee NC, Heninger GR, Price LH, Haloperidol addition in fluvoxamine-refractory obsessive-compulsive disorder: a double-blind, placebo-controlled study in patients with and without tics, *Arch Gen Psychiatry* (1994) **51**:302–8.

34 Swedo SE, Leonard HL, Trichotillomania: an obsessive-compulsive spectrum disorder? *Psychiatr Clin North Am* (1992) **15**(4):777–90.

35 Stein DJ, Hollander E, Low-dose pimozide augmentation of serotonin reuptake blockers in the treatment of trichotillomania, *J Clin Psychiatry* (1992) **53**:123–6.

36 Christenson GA, Mackenzie TB, Mitchell JE, Characteristics of 60 adult chronic hair pullers, *Am J Psychiatry* (1991) **148**:365–70.

37 Yanchick JK, Barton TL, Kelly MW, Efficacy of fluoxetine in trichotillomania, *Ann Pharmacother* (1994) **28**:1245–6.

38 Swedo SE, Leonard HL, Rapoport JL, Lenane MC, Goldberger EL, Cheslow DL, A double-blind comparison of clomipramine and desipramine in the treatment of trichotillomania, *New Engl J Med* (1989) **321**:497–500.

39 Christenson GA, Mackenzie TB, Mitchell JE, Callies AL, A placebo-controlled, double-blind crossover study of fluoxetine in trichotillomania, *Am J Psychiatry* (1991) **148**:566–71.

40 Stein DJ, Bouwer C, Hawkridge S, Emsley RA, Risperidone augmentation of serotonin reuptake inhibitors in obsessive-compulsive and related disorders, *J Clin Psychiatry* (1997) **58**(3):119–22.

41 Streichenwein SM, Thornby JI, A long-term, double-blind, placebo-controlled crossover trial of the efficacy of fluoxetine for trichotillomania, *Am J Psychiatry* (1995) **152**:1192–6.

42 Van Ameringen M, Mancini M, Oakman JM, Farvolden P, The potential role of haloperidol in the treatment of trichotillomania, *J Affect Disord* (1999) **56**:219–26.

43 Ninan PT, Knight B, Kirk L, Rothbaum BO, Kelsey G, Nemeroff CB, Beyond panic: medication effects in anxiety disorders: controlled trial of venlafaxine in trichotillomania: interim phase 1 results, *Psychopharm Bull* (1998) **34**:221–4.

44 Stahl SM, *Essential Psychopharmacology: Neuroscientific Basis and Practical Applications*, 2nd edn (Cambridge University Press: New York, 2000).

45 Mello LEAM, Villares J, Neuroanatomy of the basal ganglia, *Psychiatr Clin North Am* (1997) **10**(4):691–704.

46 Rauch SL, Savage CR, Neuroimaging and neuropsychology of the striatum, *Psychiatr Clin North Am* (1997) **10**(4):741–68.

47 Miguel EC, Rauch SL, Jenike MA, Obsessive-compulsive disorder, *Psychiatr Clin North Am* (1997) **10**(4):863–83.

48 O'Sullivan RL, Rauch SL, Breiter HC et al, Reduced basal ganglia volumes in trichotillomania measured via morphometric resonance imaging, *Biol Psychiatry* (1997) **42**:39–45.

49 Phillips KA, Kim JM, Hudson JI, Body image disturbance in body dysmorphic disorder and eating disorders. Obsessions or delusions? *Psychiatr Clin North Am* (1995) **18**(2):545–61.

50 Gamberino WC, Gold MS, Neurobiology of tobacco smoking and other addictive disorders, *Psychiatr Clin North Am* (1999) **22**(2): 301–29.

51 Hollander E, Buchalter AJ, DeCaria CM, Pathological gambling, *Psychiatr Clin North Am* (2000) **23**(3):629–41.

52 Koob GF, Neurobiology of addictions: toward the development of new therapies, *Ann NY Acad Sci* (2000) **909**:170–85.

53 Busatto GF, Kerwin RW, Schizophrenia, psychosis, and the basal ganglia, *Psychiatr Clin North Am* (1997) **10**(4):897–910.

54 Stam CJ de Bruin JP, van Haelst AM, van der Gugten J, Kalsbeck A, Influence of the mesocortical dopaminergic system on activity, food hoarding, social agonistic behavior, and spatial delayed alternation in male rats, *Behav Neurosci* (1989) **103**(1):24–35.

55 Drago F, Lissandrello CO, The 'low dose' concept and the paradoxical effects of prolactin on grooming and sexual behaviour, *Eur J Pharmacol* (2000) **405**(1–3): 131–7.

4
Unusual symptoms of OCD

Dan J Stein, Naomi Fineberg and Brian Harvey

Obsessive compulsive disorder (OCD) is in many ways one of the most homogeneous of psychiatric disorders. Patients present with characteristic symptoms of obsessions and compulsions, with concerns focusing on contamination and other kinds of possible harm. While the exact content of such symptoms may vary slightly from patient to patient (for example, obsessions with dirt, germs or bodily secretions, or having to wash hands, shampoo hair, or clean clothes), the form of symptoms (that is, the focus on contamination) appears to be universal. Even when comparing OCD in patients from vastly different cultures, the content of the symptoms seems to differ only slightly, and the form is the same.[1]

Nevertheless, during the course of treating different patients with OCD, clinicians are likely to come across symptoms that are relatively unusual. These anomalous complaints raise several interesting issues: patients with unusual OCD symptoms may present diagnostic dilemmas and be misdiagnosed; exploration of the psychobiology of the symptoms may provide new clues for understanding the pathogenesis of this disorder; and such patients may require novel adjustments to their treatment approach. In this chapter we review some unusual symptoms of OCD with a focus on these clinically relevant matters.

'Classical' OCD

Before considering some of the less common OCD symptoms, it may be useful to summarize the more typical presentations of the disorder. Table 4.1 lists common OCD symptoms documented in a large group of subjects.[2] The most common symptoms are those that involve contamination and possible harm. The possibility that procedural routines revolving around such concerns are encoded in the basal ganglia is consistent with a wealth of information suggesting that cortico–striatal–thalamic–cortical (CSTC) circuits are crucial in mediating OCD. It is also likely that such symptoms are mediated by the serotonin

Table 4.1 Classical symptoms of OCD.

Concerns about contamination → washing/cleaning rituals
Concerns about harm to self/others → checking rituals
Ordering/symmetry concerns → ordering/symmetry rituals

neurotransmitter system, which apparently has an important role in harm assessment.

Factor analyses of OCD confirm the importance of these particular symptoms. A recent study demonstrated four factors: cleanliness/washing; aggressive/sexual/religious obsessions/checking; ordering/symmetry; and hoarding.[3] Interestingly, ordering/symmetry symptoms have been associated with comorbid tics, discussed in the next section. Other sections of this chapter focus on hoarding, and on unusual somatic, sensory, stereotypic, impulsive, interpersonal and abstract symptoms. A final section looks at aspects of OCD symptoms that may be associated with failure to respond to treatment.

OCD and tics

One of the important advances in recent understanding of OCD is a recognition of the phenomenological and neurobiological overlap between OCD and Tourette's syndrome (TS). Up to 30% of patients with OCD may manifest tics, while many patients with TS may meet criteria for OCD. Even more convincingly, TS is more common than would be expected in the families of OCD probands and vice versa.[4] Recent work on an autoimmune hypothesis of OCD demonstrates that both OCD symptoms and tics may begin in the aftermath of a streptococcal infection.[5]

Interestingly, a number of symptoms are more likely to be seen in OCD patients with tics than in those without tics. In a comparison of patients with OCD and patients with both OCD and TS, the former group were more likely to have contamination obsessions and compulsions, fear of not saying the right thing, and body dysmorphic disorder; while the latter group were more likely to have an obsession with the need for symmetry accompanied by magical thinking, fear of doing something embarrassing or blurting out an obscenity, intrusive violent and/or sexual images and thoughts, touching compulsions, blinking or staring rituals, self-injurious compulsions, hoarding and counting.[6] Similarly, Holtzer and colleagues found that OCD patients with a history of tic disorder had significantly more touching, repeating, blinking, self-damaging, counting, and ordering compulsions.[7] Coprolalia, which is not uncommon in TS, is only rarely seen in OCD patients without tics.[8]

The existence of these relatively unusual OCD symptoms or of comorbid tics may reflect specific psychobiological processes that overlap with those found in TS. It has been suggested, for example, that the putamen plays a particularly important role in TS, whereas classical OCD involves the caudate (see Chapter 3).[9] Certainly, the dopamine system is likely to play a central role in TS, with dopamine-receptor antagonists constituting the treatment of choice in this disorder. Furthermore, OCD patients with tics are less likely to respond to serotonin reuptake inhibitors (SRIs) and more likely to respond to augmentation of these agents with a typical antipsychotic agent.[10]

Hoarding symptoms

Although perhaps not that uncommon in OCD, hoarding is sufficiently different to warrant mention in a separate discussion. Hoarding has been defined as the acquisition of, and failure to discard, possessions that are useless or have limited value.[11] In contradistinction to normal collecting, hoarding may be a symptom of various psychiatric disorders including OCD and obsessive-compulsive personality disorder (OCPD). The specific rationale for hoarding in OCD may vary from patient to patient, but compulsive hoarders may be characterized by a relative lack of insight.[12]

Hoarding in OCD may be associated with significant morbidity, may have specific neurobiological and psychological correlates, and may respond to pharmacotherapy or psychotherapy.[13] Of particular note is the possibility that, like comorbid tics, hoarding is a predictor of failure to respond to SRIs.[14,15] The basic neurobiology of hoarding involves dopamine, and it may be speculated that dopamine blocker augmentation is again a useful option in OCD patients where hoarding is a predominant symptom.

Unusual somatic symptoms

It has been suggested that at least a third of OCD patients have somatic concerns.[16] Contamination itself could conceivably be included under the rubric of a somatic concern, but for the purposes of the current discussion the latter term can be taken to refer primarily to obsessions or compulsions related to the appearance or health of one's body.

Excessive concern about the appearance of one's body is the hallmark of body dysmorphic disorder (BDD). There is a good deal of overlap in the phenomenology of OCD and BDD, insofar as BDD patients also have recurrent intrusive thoughts (about body appearance) and ritualistic behaviours (e.g. mirror-checking, asking for reassurance about their appearance, skin-picking). Concerns often centre on the face, breasts or buttocks, but any area of the body can be a focus of attention.[17] As in the case of OCD, insight into the excessive or irrational nature of symptoms varies from person to person. The degree to which some sufferers self-mutilate in response to their obsessions has received increased recognition recently.

Excessive concerns about the health of one's body is the defining characteristic of hypochondriasis. Once again, the phenomenology of this disorder may show considerable overlap with OCD – there are intrusive concerns which increase anxiety, followed by repetitive behaviours (e.g. reading about illness, visiting the doctor) which attempt to decrease anxiety levels.[18] Patients with OCD, in addition to their other symptoms, may worry about specific illnesses (in the past, concerns centred often on tuberculosis or cancer, now a typical concern is AIDS).

The *Diagnostic and Statistical Manual* DSM-IV rules out the diagnosis of BDD and hypochondriasis when symptoms are better explained by OCD.[19] In clinical practice, though, there are patients whose symptoms seem to fall at the intersection of these three disorders.[20] An excessive concern that one's teeth have been contaminated by an antibiotic and are pathologically yellow, for example, is one that has elements of OCD (contamination), BDD (appearance) and hypochondriasis (illness). In a patient with such a concern, and without any other obsessions or compulsions, the exact diagnosis would naturally reflect clinical judgment. The putative diagnosis of 'multiple chemical sensitivity' would also seem to lie at this intersection in some cases.

Bowel and urinary obsessions may be categorized together with somatic obsessions. Although there is again the possibility of an overlap with contamination concerns, the main focus of obsessions and compulsions in these patients is on their bowel or urinary habits or processes. Although there is little specific research on these patients,[21] standard anti-OCD interventions can be suggested.

Olfactory reference syndrome (ORS) also falls under the rubric of somatic obsessions. This term was introduced by Pryse-Phillips to differentiate non-specific concerns about personal odour, seen in a range of psychiatric disorders, from a specific condition in which such concerns were the chief characteristic.[22] Thus, patients with ORS held themselves responsible for the odour, and therefore experienced a 'contrite reaction', characterized by shame and embarrassment. Such patients 'tended to wash themselves excessively, to change their clothes with more than usual frequency, to hide themselves away, and to restrict their social and domestic excursions'. Again, there are obvious phenomenological similarities with OCD, and such patients have been reported to respond to SRIs.[23]

Interestingly, a number of 'culture-bound' syndromes also appear to revolve around somatic concerns. Koro, a condition seen in Asian countries, is characterized by concerns that the penis is shrinking. The disorder arguably meets diagnostic criteria for body dysmorphic disorder.[24] However, there are also some apparent differences between koro and BDD; for example, koro concerns may have a sudden onset, may be accompanied by panic, and may on occasion occur in epidemics. Taijin kyofusho (TKS) or anthropophobia is a condition seen in Japan, in which there is a fear of social situations. In many ways the disorder appears similar to social anxiety disorder, except that subjects are concerned less with embarrassing themselves, and more with offending others.[25] Typical symptoms in TKS include concerns about one's body odour being offensive to others. Interestingly, this disorder may respond to treatment with SRIs.[26] Thus, although TKS is unlikely to overlap entirely with either social anxiety disorder or OCD, some TKS patients may well have symptoms that are redolent of the form of these disorders.

Finally, consider 'reverse anorexia nervosa' or 'muscle dysmorphia'. Pope and colleagues used these terms to describe a hypothetical subtype of BDD characterized by pathological preoccupation with muscularity.[27,28] They suggest that this disorder may cause severe subjective distress, impaired social and occupational functioning, and abuse of anabolic steroids and other substances. Preliminary data suggest that the syndrome is far from uncommon.

Unusual sensory symptoms

Obsessions in OCD typically involve particular ideas or thoughts. However, at times obsessions primarily involve visual images, music or sounds, or the recall of past memories. In patients with Tourette's syndrome, tics may be preceded by premonitory urges, but sensory symptoms such as these are more common in TS than in OCD patients.[29]

Whereas musical hallucinations by definition have 'the compelling sense of reality of a true perception',[29] the source of which is often experienced as outside the head, in musical obsessions tunes are experienced as an internally generated cognitive product that is intrusive and inappropriate. Repetitive musical intrusions have been described after basal ganglia pathology,[30] and single photon emission computed tomography (SPECT) scanning of two patients with musical obsessions demonstrated prominent decreases of blood flow in the temporal lobes as well as frontal perfusion defects.[31] This is consistent with a literature demonstrating the involvement of the temporal lobe in normal processing of music,[32] musical hallucinations,[33] and musicogenic epilepsy.[34] Interestingly, there are case reports of obsessive musical symptoms responding to an SRI.[35]

The occasional predominance of past memories as an OCD obsession may raise the question of differential diagnosis with post-traumatic stress disorder (PTSD). In PTSD there may be intrusive memories of a traumatic event, and there may also be a certain amount of compulsive behaviour (washing after rape is not uncommon). Certainly, PTSD can potentially be misdiagnosed as OCD, and vice versa.[36] Although neurobiological research on PTSD has emphasized the role of the amygdala–hippocampus rather than cortico–striatal–thalamic–cortical (CSTC) circuits, there may nevertheless be some overlap in the psychobiology of these two disorders. Thus, the serotonin agonist methylchlorophenylpiperazine (mCPP) can exacerbate symptoms in both conditions, and it is possible that the SRIs are selectively effective in both.

Another disorder in which sensory-like symptoms occur, and which arguably also has a somatic element, is depersonalization. Here there are repetitive concerns about the reality of one's sense of self. Although classified as a dissociation disorder, such symptoms may be experienced as intrusive. There is evidence that depersonalization is mediated by the serotonin system and may respond to serotonin reuptake inhibitors.[37]

Unusual stereotypic symptoms

Stereotypic movement disorder is described in DSM-IV as characterized by repetitive, seemingly driven, but non-functional motoric behaviour that is not better accounted for by compulsions and tics.[19] Stereotypic movement disorder (SMD) should also be differentiated from the motor stereotypies (or 'punding') seen secondary to central nervous system stimulants such as amphetamine and cocaine,[38] and from perseverative symptoms secondary to various kinds of brain lesion.[39]

The stereotypies of SMD are redolent of animal stereotypies, insofar as they involve rhythmic, repeated, purposeless behaviour.[40] There is a rich animal literature demonstrating that stereotypies can be elicited reliably by physical confinement or emotional deprivation, as well as by manipulations of the dopamine and other systems. More recently, there has been increased attention to behaviour such as paw-licking in dogs (acral lick dermatitis), hair-pulling in cats (psychogenic alopecia), and feather-picking in birds, as possible analogues of OCD.[41]

In humans the line between stereotypies and compulsions is not always clearly discernible. There is the occasional OCD patient, for example, who has to sniff (sometimes in response to contamination concerns, but sometimes simply ritualistically), or who has a compulsion to blink, to swallow, or to make some other movement.[42] Also, self-injurious stereotypies such as skin-picking are not uncommon in OCD, body dysmorphic disorder, and trichotillomania.[43] Stereotypies may also overlap with tics, and perhaps even with stuttering, although they differ to the extent that they are under more complete voluntary control.

Conversely, some patients with symptoms such as head-banging or body-rocking, which might well fall under the diagnosis of stereotypic movement disorder, may describe their symptoms in a way that is very reminiscent of OCD. While some patients with self-injurious stereotypies (such as skin-picking, nail-biting, nose-picking) may describe their symptoms in terms of tension relief (so paralleling the symptoms of an impulse control disorder), others describe their symptoms as ritualistic and senseless (so approaching a compulsion).[43,44]

Unusual impulsive symptoms

Some authors have suggested that one way of looking at the OCD spectrum may be in terms of the dimension of compulsivity and impulsivity.[45–47] This perspective is based on the notion that compulsivity may reflect harm avoidance, whereas impulsivity reflects risk-seeking. Thus OCD falls at the compulsive end of an OCD spectrum, whereas impulsive disorders (e.g. pathological gambling, kleptomania, pyromania, uncontrolled buying) fall at the impulsive end, and disorders such as Tourette's syndrome, trichotillomania and obsessive-compulsive personality disorder demonstrate both compulsive and impulsive characteristics.

Nevertheless, there are patients with supposedly impulsive disorders in whom there is also apparent overlap of compulsive and impulsive symptoms. Occasionally a patient with kleptomania, for example, will describe having to steal exactly three items on each occasion. Perhaps more commonly, patients with kleptomania will hoard stolen goods in a way that is particularly reminiscent of OCD. (Conversely, of course, some patients with OCD or TS may have considerable comorbid impulsive-aggression.)

Indeed, the overlap between compulsive and impulsive aspects of symptoms is one that is often useful to consider. As noted above, self-injurious behaviours such as skin-picking may have both compulsive and impulsive features. Similar claims can arguably be made about symptoms such as trichotillomania and trichophagy,[48] and about the range of symptoms (including concerns about food contamination or difficulty in swallowing) in various eating disorders (anorexia nervosa, bulimia nervosa, pica, polydipsia).[49]

Unusual interpersonal symptoms

Jealousy may be a normal or pathological phenomenon.[50] Pathological jealousy has been divided into reactive jealousy, which appears to result from an interaction between pre-existing personality and the experience of a threat to the relationship; and symptomatic jealousy, which results from an underlying disease process.[51] Classifications of pathological jealousy have often focused on delusions. Kraft-Ebbing, for example, divided these into delusions of infidelity (where the patient's conjugal partner was under suspicion) and delusions of jealousy (when the patient's partner in an extramarital affair was under suspicion).[52] Stalking and erotomania fall within the spectrum of these conditions.

Classifications of pathological jealousy have only rarely included a category of obsessional jealousy.[53] Nevertheless, this category would appear useful insofar as jealous thoughts may be experienced as intrusive and excessive, and may lead to compulsive behaviours such as checking. Ego-dystonicity in both classical OCD symptoms and pathological jealousy varies considerably from patient to patient, and the notion of a spectrum from obsessional to delusional may therefore be useful here. Interestingly, however, both cognitive-behavioural therapy and SRIs have been reported as useful in obsessional jealousy.[54]

There is also the question of what has been termed 'compulsive' sexual behaviour. Strictly speaking this does not always fall into the 'interpersonal' category: compulsive masturbation, for example, can take place when the person is alone (although typically even this is accompanied by fantasies of the interpersonal). Furthermore, clinicians should be careful to differentiate classical obsessions with sexual content (e.g. ego-dystonic homosexual images in a heterosexual person), paraphilias, and compulsive sexual behaviour (also termed non-paraphilic sexual addiction and hypersexual disorder).[55]

Obsessive compulsive disorder often insinuates itself within an interpersonal relationship. For example, a patient may repeatedly ask a family member for reassurance, and feel relief of anxiety only upon hearing a particular phrase. When family members become active participants in the rituals, there is even the risk of a *folie à deux*.[56] Furthermore, cases of trichotillomania or body dysmorphic disorder by proxy – with symptoms focused on another – have been described. These points emphasize the clinical importance of a thorough family history, and of including significant others in the treatment plan.

Unusually abstract symptoms

In children, symptoms of OCD can be quite concrete. A child may wash repeatedly without necessarily being able to articulate a clear rationale for this behaviour. On the other hand, some adults develop symptoms of OCD that are remarkably abstract. These patients, who would perhaps at one time have been termed 'pure obsessionals', may have complex mental rituals with complex series of arguments running through their heads and justifying their current actions.

One patient of ours is particularly interesting to mention in this regard. This was a patient who during a philosophy course began to be obsessed with the idea that everything he knew or perceived might in fact be imaginary. Initially this began simply as a philosophical debate, but its persistence was felt as intrusive and senseless. In order to get rid of the thought, he felt compelled to go through a mental argument that would prove the reality of his knowledge and perceptions. This argument would take some time to complete, and until a satisfactory conclusion was reached, he felt intensely anxious. Fortunately, he responded to treatment with an SRI.

Another abstract kind of symptom is that of scrupulosity. Some of the earliest published cases of individuals with symptoms redolent of OCD described those who were concerned about their spiritual flaws, and who subsequently made ritualistic expiation. Fortunately, a growing literature arguing that such symptoms respond to standard OCD treatments is now available. Both cognitive-behavioural interventions and medication may be useful.[57]

The term 'impulsions' was employed by Bender and Schilder to describe a childhood phenomenon in which there was preoccupation with a specific subject (e.g. motor cars), leading to the performance of specific actions (e.g. painting cars).[58] These differed from obsessions and compulsions in that patients were not bothered by them. Although no longer much used, this construct remains relevant both to disorders such as Asperger's syndrome, and arguably also to concepts of subclinical OCD or obsessive compulsive personality disorder.

Unusually problematic symptoms

Some OCD patients seem to be particularly difficult to treat. This may have to do with the particular form of the presenting symptoms, with increased severity of symptoms, or with Axis I or II comorbidity. Consider, for example, patients whose obsessions and compulsions revolve around physicians – 'has the psychiatrist made an accurate diagnosis?' – or around medications – 'is this tablet contaminated?' Patients who have poor insight may refuse to come in for treatment, may not immediately be diagnosed as having OCD, and may be at risk for non-compliance. Such patients can be extremely challenging.

Lack of insight should be differentiated from the degree to which a symptom is bizarre. Of course, the whole question of what is or is not bizarre is a matter of some debate;[59] but clearly some OCD symptoms are entirely understandable (concerns about acquiring AIDS after unprotected sex), while others are less so (concerns that one has made a woman pregnant simply by looking at her); whether or not such symptoms have a different neurobiology has not to our knowledge been studied.

One OCD symptom type that may be significantly problematic is 'obsessional slowness'. Patients with obsessional slowness demonstrate pathological orderliness – having to undertake tasks in a precise and particular pattern. In the original description, 'primary obsessional slowness' was differentiated from slowness secondary to rituals.[60] However, later authors have argued that such cases can invariably be reanalysed as secondary to obsessions, compulsions or avoidance strategies.[61]

Hymas and colleagues found that patients with obsessional slowness invariably have increased neurological soft signs.[62] Slowness of thinking (bradyphrenia) and slowness of movement (bradykinesia) are symptoms of subcortical dementia, seen in disorders of the basal ganglia such as Parkinson's disease. Similarly, it might be suggested that obsessional slowness in OCD patients reflects basal ganglia damage. Perhaps this is not so much a separate group of OCD patients, as a subtype with more severe psychopathology. It has been suggested that these patients are less responsive to cognitive-behavioural therapy.[63]

In the context of disorders such as schizophrenia, OCD is problematic insofar as there may be accompanying loss of insight by the patient, or underdiagnosis by the clinician. Obsessive compulsive disorder is not uncommon in borderline personality disorder, and the combination of disorders may be associated with a poorer response to treatment. The extent to which OCD can be precipitated by childhood trauma has not received a great deal of attention, and perhaps deserves more. The disorder may also be seen during pregnancy, or secondary to various medical conditions; such circumstances demand an adaptation of usual treatments.

Conclusion

Although many patients with OCD present with 'classical' symptoms, a range of other, more unusual symptoms may also be seen. Some of these symptoms may unfortunately lead to delayed diagnosis, and others may interfere with treatment. It is important for clinicians to be aware of the range of unusual presentations of OCD to maximize appropriate diagnosis and early intervention.

An examination of more unusual symptoms may raise questions about current nosology. Although it is important not to oversimplify the construct of an OCD spectrum, the apparently close relationship between OCD, BDD and hypochondriasis certainly raises questions for future investigation about possible overlaps in the psychobiology of these disorders. A putative OCD spectrum of disorders may include conditions that have been considered 'culture-bound'.

It is remarkable that classical OCD, more unusual OCD symptoms, and some of the putative OCD spectrum disorders appear to respond selectively to the SRIs.[64] Further study of patients with more unusual symptoms may ultimately shed additional light on the psychobiology of OCD. The failure of patients with hoarding or with comorbid tics, for example, to respond to SRIs, points to the involvement of other neurotransmitter systems and suggests alternative routes of clinical intervention and future investigation.

Acknowledgement

Professors Stein and Harvey are supported by the Medical Research Council of South Africa.

References

1 Stein DJ, Rapoport JL, Cross-cultural studies and obsessive-compulsive disorder, *CNS Spectr* (1996) **1**:42–6.

2 Rassmussen SA, Eisen JL, Epidemiological and clinical features of obsessive-compulsive disorder. In: Jenike MA, Baer LB, Minichiello WE, eds, *Obsessive-Compulsive Disorders: Theory and Management*, 2nd edn (Year Book: Chicago, 1990).

3 Leckman JF, Grice DE, Boardman J et al, Symptoms of obsessive-compulsive disorder, *Am J Psychiatry* (1997) **154**: 911–17.

4 Pauls DL, Towbin KE, Leckman JF et al, Gilles de la Tourette's syndrome and obsessive compulsive disorder: evidence supporting a genetic relationship, *Arch Gen Psychiatry* (1986) **43**: 1180–2.

5 Swedo SE, Leonard HL, Garvey M et al, Pediatric autoimmune neuropsychiatric disorders associated with streptococcal infections: clinical description of the first 50 cases, *Am J Psychiatry* (1998) **155**:264–71.

6 George MS, Trimble MR, Ring HA et al, Obsessions in obsessive-compulsive disorder with and without Gilles de la Tourette's syndrome, *Am J Psychiatry* (1992) **150**:93–7.

7 Holtzer JC, Price LH, McDougle CJ et al, Obsessive compulsive disorder with and without a chronic tic disorder: a comparison of symptoms in 70 patients, *Br J Psychiatry* (1994) **164**: 469–73.

8 Pitman RK, Jenike MA, Coprolalia in obsessive-compulsive disorder: a missing link, *J Nerv Ment Dis* (1988) **176**:311–13.

9 Rauch SL, Baxter LR, Neuroimaging in obsessive-compulsive disorder and related disorders. In: Jenicke MA, Baer L, Minichiello WE, eds, *Obsessive-Compulsive Disorders: Practical Management*, 3rd edn (Mosby: St Louis, 1998).

10 McDougle CJ, Goodman WK, Leckman JF et al, Haloperidol addition in fluvoxamine-refractory obsessive-compulsive disorder: a double-blind placebo-controlled study in patients with and without tics, *Arch Gen Psychiatry* (1994) **51**:302–8.

11 Frost RO, Gross RC, The hoarding of possessions, *Behav Res Ther* (1993) **31**:367–81.

12 Greenberg D, Compulsive hoarding, *Am J Psychother* (1987) **41**: 409–16.

13 Stein DJ, Seedat S, Potocnik F, Hoarding: a review, *Isr J Psychiatry* (1999) **36**:35–46.

14 Black DW, Monahan P, Gable J et

al, Hoarding and treatment response in 38 nondepressed subjects with obsessive-compulsive disorder, *J Clin Psychiatry* (1998) **59**:420–5.

15 Mataix-Cols D, Rauch SL, Manzo PA, Jenike MA, Baer L, Use of factor-analyzed symptom dimensions to predict outcome with serotonin reuptake inhibitors and placebo in the treatment of obsessive-compulsive disorder, *Am J Psychiatry* (1999) **156**: 1409–16.

16 Simeon D, Hollander E, Stein DJ, Cohen LJ, Aronowitz B, Body dysmorphic disorder in the DSM-IV field trial for obsessive-compulsive disorder, *Am J Psychiatry* (1995) **152**:1207–9.

17 Phillips KA, McElroy SL, Keck PE, Pope HG, Hudson JI, Body dysmorphic disorder: 30 cases of imagined ugliness, *Am J Psychiatry* (1993) **150**:302–8.

18 Fallon BA, Schneier FR, Marshall R et al, The pharmacotherapy of hypochondriasis, *Psychopharmacol Bull* (1996) **32**:607–11.

19 American Psychiatric Association, *Diagnostic and Statistical Manual of Mental Disorders*, 4th edn (APA: Washington, 1994).

20 Josephson SC, Hollander E, Fallon B, Stein DJ, Obsessive-compulsive disorder, body dysmorphic disorder, and hypochondriasis: three variations on a theme, *CNS Spectr* (1996) **1**:24–31.

21 Jenike MA, Vitagliano HL, Rabinowitz J et al, Bowel obsessions responsive to tricyclic antidepressants in four patients, *Am J Psychiatry* (1987) **144**:1347–8.

22 Pryse-Phillips W, An olfactory reference syndrome, *Acta Psychiat Scand* (1971) **47**:484–509.

23 Stein DJ, Le Roux L, Bouwer C, van Heerden B, Is olfactory reference syndrome on the obsessive-compulsive spectrum? Two cases and a discussion, *J Neuropsych Clin Neurosci* (1998) **10**:96–9.

24 Stein DJ, Frenkel M, Hollander E, Classification of Koro, *Am J Psychiatry* (1991) **148**:1279–80.

25 Kleinknecht RA, Dinnel DL, Tanouye-Wilson S, Lonner WJ, Cultural variation in social anxiety and phobia: a study of Taijin Kyofusho, *Behav Ther* (1994) **17**:175–8.

26 Matsunaga H, Kiriike N, Matsui T, Iwasaki Y, Nagata T, Stein DJ, Taijin Kyofusho: a form of social anxiety disorder that responds to serotonin reuptake inhibitors? *Int J Neuropsychopharmacol*, in press.

27 Pope HG, Katz DL, Hudson JI, Anorexia nervosa and 'reverse anorexia' among 108 male bodybuilders, *Compr Psychiatry* (1993) **34**:406–9.

28 Pope HG, Gruber AJ, Choi P et al, Muscle dysmorphia, *Psychosomatics* (1997) **38**:548–57.

29 Miguel EC, do Rosario Campos MC, Prado HS et al, Sensory phenomena in obsessive-compulsive disorder and Tourette's disorder, *J Clin Psychiatry* (2000) **61**: 150–6.

30 Wodarz N, Becker T, Deckert J, Musical hallucinations associated with post thyroidectomy hypoparathyroidism and symmetric basal ganglia calcifications, *J Neurol Neurosurg Psych* (1995) **58**:763–4.

31 Zungu-Dirwayi M, Hugo F, van Heerden B, Stein DJ, Are musical obsessions a temporal lobe phenomenon? *J Neuropsych Clin Neurosci* (1999) **11**:398–400.

32 Lechevalier B, Platel H, Eustache F, Neuropsychology of musical identification, *Rev Neurol (Paris)* (1995) **151**:505–10.

33 Berrios GE, Musical hallucinations: a historical and clinical

study, *Br J Psychiatry* (1990) **156**:188–94.

34 Wieser HG, Hungerbuhler H, Siegel AM, Buck A, Musicogenic epilepsy: review of the literature and case report with ictal single photon emission tomography, *Epilepsia* (1997) **38**:200–7.

35 Cameron OG, Wasielewski P, Clomipramine treatment of possible atypical obsessive-compulsive disorder, *J Clin Psychopharmacol* (1990) **10**: 375–6.

36 Pitman RK, Posttraumatic obsessive-compulsive disorder: a case study, *Compr Psychiatry* (1993) **34**:102–7.

37 Hollander E, Liebowitz MR, DeCaria M et al, Treatment of depersonalization with serotonin reuptake blockers, *J Clin Psychopharmacol* (1990) **10**:200–3.

38 Schiorring E, Psychopathology induced by 'speed drugs', *Pharmacol Biochem Behav* (1981) **14**S1:109–22.

39 Ames D, Cummings JL, Wirshing WC et al, Repetitive and compulsive behavior in frontal lobe degenerations, *J Neuropsych Clin Neurosci* (1994) **6**:100–13.

40 Ridley RM, The psychology of perseverative and stereotyped behavior, *Prog Neurobiol* (1994) **44**:221–31.

41 Dodman N, Moon A, Stein DJ, Animal models of obsessive-compulsive disorder. In: Hollander E, Stein DJ, eds, *Obsessive-Compulsive Disorders: Etiology, Diagnosis, Treatment* (Marcel Dekker: New York, 1997).

42 Zella SJ, Geenens DL, Horst JN. Repetitive eructation as a manifestation of obsessive-compulsive disorder, *Psychosomatics* (1998) **39**:299–301.

43 Stein DJ, Niehaus DJH, Seedat S, Emsley RA, Phenomenology of stereotypic movement disorder, *Psychiatr Ann* (1998) **28**:307–12.

44 Jefferson JW, Thompson TD, Rhinotillexomania: psychiatric disorder or habit? *J Clin Psychiatry* (1995) **56**:56–9.

45 Stein DJ, Hollander E, The spectrum of obsessive-compulsive related disorders. In Hollander E (ed.) *Obsessive-Compulsive Related Disorders* (American Psychiatric Press: Washington, 1993).

46 Stein DJ, Hollander E, Impulsive aggression and obsessive-compulsive disorder, *Psychiatr Ann* (1993) **23**:389–95.

47 McElroy SL, Phillips KA, Keck PE, Obsessive-compulsive spectrum disorders, *J Clin Psychiatry* (1994) **55**:33–51.

48 Bouwer C, Stein DJ, Trichobezoars in trichotillomania: case report and literature review, *Psychosom Med* (1998) **60**:658–60.

49 Stein DJ, Bouwer C, Van Heerden B, Pica and the obsessive-compulsive spectrum disorders, *S Afr J Psychiatry* (1996) **86**: 1586–92.

50 Shepard M, Morbid jealousy: some clinical and social aspects of a psychiatric symptom, *J Ment Sci* (1961) **107**:687–753.

51 White GK, Mullen PE, *Jealousy: Theory, Research and Clinical Strategies* (Guildford: New York, 1989).

52 Kraft-Ebbing R von, Ueber Eifersuchtswahn beim Manne, *J Psychiat Neurol* (1892) **10**:212–31.

53 Mooney HB, Pathological jealousy and psychochemotherapy, *Br J Psychiatry* (1965) **111**:1023–42.

54 Stein DJ, Hollander E, Serotonin reuptake blockers for the treatment of obsessional jealousy, *J Clin Psychiatry* (1994) **55**:30–3.

55 Stein DJ, Black DW, Pienaar W, Sexual disorders not otherwise specified: Compulsive, impulsive or addictive? *CNS Spectr* (2000)

5(1):60–4.

56   Torch EM, Shared obsessive-compulsive disorder in a married couple: a new variant of folie a deux? *J Clin Psychiatry* (1996) **57**:489.

57   Fallon BA, Liebowitz MR, Hollander E et al, The pharmacotherapy of moral or religious scrupulosity, *J Clin Psychiatry* (1990) **51**: 517–21.

58   Bender L, Schilder P, Impulsions: a specific disorder of the behavior of children, *Arch Neurol Psychiat* (1940) **44**:990–1008.

59   Spitzer RL, First MB, Kendler KS, Stein DJ, The reliability of three definitions of bizarre delusions, *Am J Psychiatry* (1993) **150**: 880–4.

60   Rachman SJ, Primary obsessional slowness, *Behav Res Ther* (1974) **12**:9–18.

61   Veale D, Classification and treatment of obsessional slowness, *Br J Psychiatry* (1993) **162**:198–203.

62   Hymas N, Lees A, Bolton D et al, The neurology of obsessional slowness, *Brain* (1991) **114**: 2203–33.

63   Clark DA, Sugrim I, Bolton D, Primary obsessional slowness: a nursing treatment programme and a 13 year old male adolescent, *Behav Res Ther* (1982) **20**: 289–92.

64   Stein DJ, Advances in the neurobiology of obsessive-compulsive disorder: Implications for conceptualizing putative obsessive-compulsive and spectrum disorders, *Psychiatr Clin North Am* (2000) **23**:545–62.

5

Obsessive compulsive disorder and quality of life

Lorrin M Koran

The quality of a person's life cannot be captured simply. Life is too multifaceted, and each facet's value is not universally agreed. Moreover, no simple metric exists for adding or subtracting one facet's value to that of another. Nonetheless, policy-makers, health-care payers and physicians have become interested in measuring the impact of medical interventions not only on the symptoms of a disease or disorder, but also on the quality of the patient's life. The crassest motives are economic: to carve out a niche in the medical marketplace by arguing that larger effects on some aspect of quality of life justify the selection of a particular treatment. More defensible motives are humanitarian: to find those treatments that bring the broadest and largest benefits to the patient.

Physicians attempt to quantify medicine's contribution to patients' health-related quality of life (HRQL) in their role as advocates for the whole person, and in response to the increasing political scrutiny of the high costs of medical services and technologies. The 1990s saw the publication of hundreds of studies concerning numerous diseases and the creation of a specialized journal, *Quality of Life Research*, to communicate research findings. However, the study of health-related quality of life is still a young discipline, and the portion devoted to obsessive compulsive disorder (OCD) is in its infancy.

Attempts to measure 'quality of life' have brought the realization that the concept is not only multifaceted, but also culturally bound. To allow collaborative research across national boundaries, expert panels have helped the World Health Organization create a quality of life assessment questionnaire that is valid cross-culturally.[1] The six broad domains of this thoughtfully designed questionnaire have conceptual appeal: these domains are physical; psychological; level of independence; social relationships; environment; and spirituality/religion/personal beliefs. Of course, many other conceptual schemes have been used.[2,3] Thus, this chapter's summary of information concerning HRQL in adults with OCD is constrained by having to draw on studies using disparate methodologies.

Relationships between OCD and quality of life

The five studies that have examined aspects of HRQL in individuals with OCD are all limited by ascertainment bias, and most suffer from small sample size and questions about the construct validity of the assessment instruments. These methodological limitations require us to view the results with caution. Moreover, results describing individuals attending for treatment of OCD should not be generalized to individuals with OCD in the community who have not sought care, since their condition may be milder or more likely to be transient or episodic.[4,5] The reverse is also true.

An early study of HRQL in OCD involved a survey of 200 members of the Obsessive-Compulsive Disorder Association of South Africa by means of a detailed self-report questionnaire.[6] Seventy-five questionnaires were returned (37.5% of those mailed), of which 39 reported OCD symptoms and the remainder only noted hair-pulling. The individuals with OCD had a mean age of 33.4 years (sD 14.5, range 11–68 years) and about half were female. All but one were white, and of the adults, 15 (44%) were married, 2 (6%) were widowed and 17 (50%) were single.

The respondent's HRQL was impaired in many domains. More than half reported that OCD caused moderate or severe interference with socializing, family relationships and ability to study; 30% reported moderate or severe interference with ability to work. A little less than half reported that their current obsessions or compulsions caused moderate or severe distress. Three-quarters had decreased self-esteem and half had thought about suicide.

A similar questionnaire survey, albeit of a much larger sample, was conducted among members of the Obsessive Compulsive Foundation, a US patient advocacy, education and lobbying organization.[7] The investigators surveyed every fourth member and received responses from about one-quarter (26.9%) of those surveyed (701 of 2670). The respondents had a mean age of 37 years (sD 14, range 5–82 years). Parents, guardians or close relatives completed young children's questionnaires. A little more than half the respondents (55%) were women, and the majority (95%) were white.

The pattern of impairment of HRQL domains closely resembled the pattern described in South Africa. The OCD had interfered with the social and work functioning of more than half the respondents, and for nearly two-thirds it had interfered with their socializing or making friends; OCD caused difficulties in family relationships for almost three-quarters of the respondents. Among those previously employed, OCD had prevented about 40% of respondents working, in many cases for more than a year. About 20% of the respondents received disability income payments when unemployed, substantiating the direct social costs as well as the personal costs of the disorder. Impaired vocational functioning was suggested by the observation that the respondents' average career achievement did not match their educational attainment, i.e. the respondents' mean income resembled that of the general population despite their much higher level of education (college degrees, 40% versus 14.7%, and postgraduate degrees, 18% versus 7.5%).[8]

The HRQL domain of general wellbeing was usually diminished: obsessions caused moderate to severe distress for 59% of respondents and compulsions brought these distress levels to 51%. Moreover, lowered self-esteem was present in more than 90%, thoughts of suicide had bothered more than half, and one-eighth had been led to a suicide attempt. Reduced wellbeing was also reflected in the abuse of alcohol (reported by 18%) and of other drugs (13%).

Only one study has compared OCD patients' HRQL to norms for the general population and for individuals with another chronic disorder. Koran and his colleagues studied 60 medication-free outpatients with moderate to severe OCD who were enrolling in a medication trial.[9] The comparison norms were established in an independent study,[10] which limits but does not invalidate the comparisons. The HRQL was assayed with the Medical Outcomes Study 36-item Short-Form Health Survey (SF-36), a self-report questionnaire.[11] The SF-36 generates measures of physical domains of HRQL (physical functioning; role limitations due to physical health; and bodily pain), mental health domains (mental health, reflecting primarily anxiety and depression; role limitations due to emotional symptoms; and social functioning) and measures of 'general health' and 'vitality' (or energy).

Of the 60 subjects, 26 (43%) were women. The patients' mean age was 40.1 years (SD 10.6, range 19–67 years). Thirty patients (50%) were married, 8 (13%) divorced and 22 (37%) were single.

The investigators' hypothesis that OCD would most affect social relationships and instrumental role functioning (functioning in work, school and homemaking) was confirmed: the subjects' median scores for role limitations due to emotional problems, social functioning and mental health all fell below the 25th percentile for the US general population. In contrast, the subjects' median scores for the physical health domains were at or above the general population medians. Greater severity of OCD, as measured by the Yale–Brown Obsessive Compulsive Scale (Y-BOCS, see Appendix 1, p. 183)[12] was associated with poorer social functioning, but not with role limitations due to emotional problems, even after controlling for depression severity at baseline (as measured by the Hamilton Depression Rating Scale).[13] The absence of a relationship between OCD severity and role limitations may reflect this scale's limited range and variance (raw score from 3 to 6) or the absence of extremely severe OCD cases in the study group. Alternatively, the absence of a relationship may have resulted from some patients' ability to exert more control over their symptoms at work or school than at home.

Unemployment was higher in the study group than in the US general population (22% versus 9%) and 9 of the 13 unemployed subjects attributed their unemployment to the effects of OCD. Unlike the Obsessive Compulsive Foundation survey respondents, many of whom were not in treatment,[7] these volunteers for a medication trial did not differ substantially from the general US population in history of alcohol abuse (15% versus 11%) or of suicide attempts (3% versus 2%).[14] As one would expect, the median scores of the OCD subjects were higher than those of patients with type 2 diabetes on all SF-36 physical health domains, and lower on all mental health domains.

Although suggesting that OCD is associated with lower HRQL in certain domains, this study was limited by ascertainment bias (volunteers for a medication trial who had to meet strict inclusion and exclusion criteria) and by a relatively small sample size. In addition, the proportion of women was greater in the study group than in the comparison groups, which increased the differences in SF-36 scores. Finally, the validity of the SF-36 in measuring HRQL in subjects with OCD has not been established; many researchers prefer disorder-specific measurement tools.

Although many treatments are effective in relieving OCD symptoms,[15] we know very little about how successful treatment affects the HRQL of patients. Bystritsky and his colleagues have conducted the only study in this area, examining change in HRQL in 30 consecutive, treatment-resistant OCD patients after 6 weeks of treatment in a partial hospitalization program.[16] The patients' mean age was 34 years (range 18–56 years) and two-thirds were men. Only 13% were married. The investigators used Lehman's Quality of Life scale, which was developed to measure HRQL in patients with schizophrenia.[3] The scale provides objective and subjective (patient satisfaction) measures of activities, health, safety, living situation and of functioning related to family, social roles, work and finances. After treatment, patient interviews indicated significant changes in the objective measures reflecting activities, health and social functioning and all of the subjective measures except family functioning. The changes in quality of life showed little correlation with changes in the patients' OCD severity (Y-BOCS scores), suggesting that treatment effects on symptoms and on HRQL domains are not closely related. Further studies with larger samples, appropriate control groups, different HRQL measures and evaluation at varying time points are indicated.

Socioeconomic effects of OCD

The economic costs of OCD have been estimated in two studies. Dupont and colleagues used a human capital methodology to estimate direct and indirect costs of OCD in the USA.[17] Taking lifetime prevalence data from the Epidemiological Catchment Area (ECA) study,[18] they estimated that reduced or lost economic productivity for individuals affected by OCD was $5.9 billion in 1990, or 70.4% of OCD's total economic cost. They also estimated a 2% suicide rate for individuals with OCD, resulting in a 1990 loss to the US economy of $255 million. This 2% estimate may be low. In a separate analysis of the ECA data, Hollander and his colleagues[19] found that individuals with comorbid OCD (OCD accompanied by other psychiatric disorders) had a 15% rate of suicide attempts, while those with uncomplicated OCD had a rate of 3.6%. Extrapolating the proportion of attempts that would be repeated over a lifetime and result in eventual success cannot, of course, be done with much precision.

Leon and colleagues derived other measures of the OCD's social costs from the ECA data.[20] They found higher unemployment rates in adult men with OCD compared to individuals with no Axis I disorder (45% versus 20%); the proportion of individuals who had been unemployed for at least 5 years was much higher (18% versus 5%). Unemployment rates for women with OCD were also elevated, but less dramatically. Individuals with OCD were receiving disability payments at far higher rates than individuals with no Axis I disorder (23% versus 5% for men, and 13% versus 4% for women).

Impact of OCD on marital relationships and the family

Most studies,[7,21–23] but not all,[9] have found that patients with OCD have lower marriage rates than the general population (80.6% for women, 73.2% for men).[24] In the ECA survey data, individuals with OCD had higher rates of divorce and separation than individuals without OCD.[2] Whether the severity of OCD symptoms or particular symptom patterns such as hoarding or religious obsessions have a greater impact on marriage rates has not been determined. Marital maladjustment or dissatisfaction has been reported in nearly half of married OCD sufferers.[25,26] Only large-scale, controlled studies can determine whether these rates are higher than those in the general population. One study suggests they may not be.[27]

In my experience, OCD often diminishes the quality of family relationships. The person with the disorder may ask family members, for example, to avoid 'contaminated' objects or furniture in the home or to shower and wash all clothes after exposure to 'contaminated' outside areas, to aid in checking that all the doors and windows are locked and that all appliances have been unplugged before going to bed each night, or to provide repeated reassurances that no dangerous situation exists. The patient may forbid family members to use a bathroom or may fill the house with hoarded items so that most rooms become unusable.[28–30] If family members fail to comply with these demands, the patient may erupt in anger or intense anxiety and subject the family to very unpleasant verbal abuse. Family members, especially parents, may blame themselves for the disorder, or feel guilty if their behavior increases the sufferer's anxiety or depression.

Despite their methodological limitations, the studies of the impact of OCD on family relationships and family members all report a substantial adverse effect. In a survey of 419 Obsessive Compulsive Foundation members, 73% reported interference with family relationships.[31] Nearly all family members (85%) were bothered by the respondent's OCD rituals.[32] In a study using a semistructured interview to evaluate the accommodation to OCD by the family members of 34 OCD patients, more than one-third of the family members had modified family routines because of the patient's symptoms and more than half reported that accommodating to these symptoms had caused at least moderately intense distress.[28]

More detail is provided by a study of 19 families with an adult member with OCD, but the small sample size necessitates caution in viewing the results.[33] Disrupted family and social life was reported by more than half of spouses, and anger and frustration, family conflicts, the patient's depression and marital difficulties disturbed nearly half. More than one-third mentioned sexual difficulties, guilt and fatigue. Compared with well-matched control families, the OCD families had lower scores on all seven scales of a family assessment measure (problem-solving, communication, roles, behavior control, affective responsiveness, affective involvement and general functioning). The OCD families scored in the 'unhealthy' range significantly more often on scales measuring communication, affective involvement and general functioning.

Another study of the family burden of OCD utilized structured interviews with 32 key relatives (primarily spouses or parents) of 32 adult patients with OCD.[34] Moderate or severe burden was reported by more than one-third in the form of (for example) difficulty taking trips or holidays, poor social relationships (due entirely to the patient's difficulties, in half of those interviewed) and neglect of hobbies. More than half of the relatives cited 'Feeling of having given up leading one's life as wanted' (58%), 'Feeling of not being able to stand the situation any longer' (68%), and 'crying or depressive feelings' (84%). The authors concluded that OCD imposes a family burden similar to that imposed by major depression or schizophrenia.

How treatment of OCD affects the quality of life of patients' family members has not been studied. However, a study by Emmelkamp and colleagues suggests some benefit.[25] Treatment reduced the partners' anxiety, anger and marital dissatisfaction.

The detrimental effects of OCD on family relationships and social role functioning may create negative feedback loops. For example, sufferers' rates of help-seeking and degree of cooperation with treatment could be adversely affected by poor interpersonal and familial relationships or impaired ability to meet social role responsibilities. The resulting absent or inadequate treatment would perpetuate the illness. Conversely, family education, family support groups and participation in the patient's treatment may increase the likelihood of a favorable outcome. The fragmentary data available are consistent with these hypotheses.[29,35,36]

Considerations for future research

Because little is known, there is much yet to learn. Future studies could profitably investigate:

- The effects of OCD on HRQL in large samples of affected individuals. Patients in treatment should be distinguished from individuals in the community with OCD, since many of those who have not sought treatment may have milder forms of the disorder.[4,5]
- How the effects of OCD on HRQL vary with patients' gender, age at onset, symptom severity, symptom type (e.g. obsessions only, obsessions and compulsions, hoarding versus cleaning versus checking to prevent terrible consequences), and comorbid psychiatric conditions. For example, the effects on women, who are frequently expected to fulfill homemaking or mothering roles, may well differ from those on men, who are usually expected to enter the workforce. Individuals whose developmental years were substantially affected by the presence of OCD may exhibit different HRQL effects than those whose OCD began in adulthood. Individuals with obsessions only may have been more successful in hiding their disorder, with lesser effects on some HRQL domains.
- The degree to which pharmacotherapies and cognitive-behavioral therapies reverse adverse effects of OCD on particular domains of HRQL. Is combined therapy more effective with regard to any domains? How quickly does treatment reverse OCD's adverse effects on HRQL? One would expect symptoms to improve sooner than interpersonal relationships and vocational performance, for example.
- The costs of attaining various degrees of improvement in HRQL domains, as incurred by the affected individual, the family, the individual's health plan and society at large. Once costs to the interested parties have been identified, they can be weighed against the benefits each party reaps. Placing an economic value on many HRQL benefits, however, will require input from several disciplines since they have no widely agreed monetary value.

Methodological considerations

The HRQL instruments that deserve serious consideration in future studies include the SF-36, Lehman's Quality of Life scale and others that have been commonly used and validated in other populations: the EuroQol,[37] WHOQOL,[1] Nottingham Health Profile,[38,39] Quality of Well-Being Scale,[26] the Social Adjustment Scale,[40] and the five-item Work and Social Adjustment Scale. The last-mentioned scale can be administered by interactive telephone technology.[41] The relative advantages and disadvantages of these measures will vary with each study's budget and aims.

In planning any study, attention to certain methodological questions will enhance the value of the results. Experienced investigators recommend attending to the assessor's skill level (health-care professional, social scientist or trained observer); who the respondent is (the patient, a family member or another informant); the quality of life domains to be assessed; the assessment method (interview, questionnaire or diary); whether to use generic or disease-specific instruments; the time-frame encompassed; and the reliability, validity and sensitivity of the measures utilized.[42] These issues and findings with regard to other mental disorders are discussed elsewhere.[2,43]

Conclusion

The available data suggest that OCD substantially and adversely affects the HRQL of sufferers and their families. Even in the absence of a consensus regarding how to conceptualize or measure HRQL, studies should be designed to further delineate and quantify the suffering and impairment associated with OCD and the costs, benefits and limitations of treatment.

References

1   Skevington SM, Bradshaw J, Saxena S, Selecting national items for the WHOQOL: Conceptual and psychometric considerations, *Soc Sci Med* (1999) **48**:473–87.

2   Katschnig H, Freeman H, Sartorius N, *Quality of Life in Mental Disorders*. (John Wiley: Chichester, 1997).

3   Lehman AF, Measurement of quality of life among persons with severe and persistent mental disorders, *Soc Psych Psychiatr Epidemiol* (1996) **31**:78–88.

4   Nelson E, Rice J, Stability of diagnosis of obsessive-compulsive disorder in the epidemiological catchment area study, *Am J Psychiatry* (1997) **154**:826–31.

5   Degonda M, Wyss M, Angst J, The Zurich Study XVIII. Obsessive-compulsive disorders and syndromes in the general population, *Eur Arch Psych Clin Neurosci* (1993) **243**:16–22.

6   Stein DJ, Roberts M, Hollander E et al, Quality of life and pharmaco-economic aspects of obsessive-compulsive disorder. A South African survey, *S Afr Med J* (1996) **8**(suppl. 12): 1579–85.

7   Hollander E, Stein D, Kwon JH et al, Psychosocial function and economic costs of obsessive-compulsive disorder, *CNS Spectrums* (1997) **2**:16–25.

8   US Bureau of Census, *Statistical Abstract of the United States: 1995*, 115th edn (US Government Printing Office: Washington DC, 1995).

9   Koran LM, Thienemann ML, Davenport R, Quality of life for patients with obsessive-compulsive disorder, *Am J Psychiatry* (1996) **153**:783–8.

10 Ware JE, Snow KK, Kosinski M et al, *SF-36 Health Survey Manual and Interpretation Guide* (New England Medical Center, Health Institute: Boston, 1993).

11 McHorney CA, Ware JE, Raczek AE, The MOS 36-item Short-Form Health Survey (SF-36). II: Psychometric and clinical tests of validity in measuring physical and mental health constructs, *Med Care* (1993) **31**:247–63.

12 Goodman WK, Price LH, Rasmussen SA et al, The Yale-Brown Obsessive Compulsive Scale, I: development, use, and reliability, *Arch Gen Psychiatry* (1989) **46**:1006–11.

13 Hamilton M, Development of a rating scale for primary depressive illness, *Br J Soc Clin Psychol* (1967) **6**:278–96.

14 Markowitz JS, Weissman MM, Ouellette R, Quality of life in panic disorder, *Arch Gen Psychiatry* (1989) **46**:984–92.

15 Koran LM, Obsessive-compulsive disorder. In: *Obsessive-Compulsive and Related Disorders in Adults: A Comprehensive Clinical Guide* (Cambridge University Press: Cambridge, 1999).

16 Bystritsky A, Saxena S, Maidment K et al, Quality-of-life changes among patients with obsessive-compulsive disorder in a partial hospitalization program, *Psychiat Serv* (1999) **50**:412–14.

17 Dupont RL, Rice DP, Shiraki S et al, Economic costs of obsessive-compulsive disorder, *Med Interf* (1995) **8**:102–9.

18 Karno M, Golding JM, Sorenson SB et al, The epidemiology of obsessive-compulsive disorder in five US communities, *Arch Gen Psychiatry* (1988) **45**:1094–9.

19 Hollander E, Greenwald S, Neville D et al, Uncomplicated and comorbid obsessive-compulsive disorder in an epidemiologic sample, *Depress Anx* (1996/1997) **4**:111–19.

20 Leon AC, Portera L, Weissman MM, The social costs of anxiety disorders, *Br J Psychiatry* (1995) **166**(suppl. 27):19–22.

21. Hafner RJ, Anxiety disorders. In: Falloon IRH, ed., *Handbook of Behavioral Family Therapy* (Guilford Press: New York 1988), 203–30.

22 Stecketee G, Social support and treatment outcome of obsessive compulsive disorder at 9-month follow-up, *Behav Psychother* (1993) **21**:81–95.

23 Steketee G, Grayson JB, Foa EB, Obsessive-compulsive disorder: differences between washers and checkers, *Behav Res Ther* (1985) **23**:197–201.

24 US Bureau of Census, *Statistical Abstract of the United States: 1996*, 116th edn. (US Government Printing Office: Washington DC, 1996).

25 Emmelkamp PMG, de Haan E, Hoogduin CAL, Marital adjustment and obsessive-compulsive disorder, *Br J Psychiatry* (1990) **156**:55–60.

26 Pyne JM, Patterson TL, Kaplan RM et al, Assessment of the quality of life of patients with major depression, *Psych Serv* (1997) **48**:224–30.

27 Balslev-Olesen T, Geert-Jorgensen E, The prognosis of obsessive-compulsive disorder, *Acta Psychiatr Scand* (1989) **34**:232–41.

28 Calvocoressi L, Lewis B, Harris M et al, Family accommodation in obsessive-compulsive disorder, *Am J Psychiatry* (1995) **152**: 441–3.

29 Mehta M, A comparative study of family-based and patient-based behavioural management in obsessive-compulsive disorder, *Br J Psychiatry* (1990) **157**:133–5.

30 Shafran R, Ralph J, Tallis F, Obsessive-compulsive symptoms and the family, *Bull Menninger Clin* (1995) **59**:472–9.

31 Hollander E, Kwon K, Won JH et al, Obsessive-compulsive and spectrum disorders: overview and quality of life issues, *J Clin Psychiatry* (1996) **57**(suppl. 8):3–6.

32 Black DW, Gaffney G, Schlosser S et al, The impact of obsessive-compulsive disorder on the family: preliminary findings, *J Nerv Ment Dis* (1998) **186**:440–2.

33 Cooper M, Report on the findings of study of OCD family members, *OCD Newsl* (1994) **8**:1–2.

34 Magliano L, Tosini P, Guarneri M et al, Burden on the families of patients with obsessive-compulsive disorder: A pilot study. *Eur Psychiatry* (1996) **11**:192–7.

35 Leonard HL, Swedo SE, Lenane MC et al, A 2- to 7-year follow-up study of 54 obsessive-compulsive children and adolescents, *Arch Gen Psychiatry* (1993) **50**:429–39.

36 Steketee G, Pruyn NA, Families of individuals with obsessive-compulsive disorder. In: Swinson RP, Antony MM, Rachman S et al, eds, *Obsessive Compulsive Disorder: Theory, Research, and Treatment*, (Guilford Press: New York, 1998), 120–40.

37 Johnson JA, Coons SJ, Ergo A et al, Valuation of EuroQOL (EQ-5D) health states in an adult US sample, *Pharmacoeconomics* (1998) **13**:421–33.

38 Hunt SM, McKenna SP, McEwen J et al, The Nottingham Health profile: subjective health status and medical consultations, *Soc Sci Med* (1981) **15A**:221–9.

39 Lukkarinen H, Hentinen M, Assessment of quality of life with the Nottingham Health Profile among women with coronary artery disease, *Heart Lung* (1998) **27**:189–99.

40 Weissman MM, Prusoff BA, Thompson WD et al, Social adjustment by self-report in a community sample and in psychiatric outpatients, *J Nerv Ment Dis* (1978) **166**:317–26.

41 Mundt JC, Kobak KA, Greist JH et al, *Work and social adjustment scale: an alternative quality-of-life instrument.* Poster presented at the 39th Annual NCDEU Meeting, Boca Raton, FL, 1–4 June 1999.

42 Aaronson NK, Quality of life assessment in clinical trials: methodologic issues, *Control Clin Trials* (1989) **10**:195-208S.

43 Gladis MM, Gosch EA, Dishuk NM et al, Quality of life: expanding the scope of clinical significance, *J Consult Clin Psychol* (1999) **67**:320–31.

6
The role of genetic factors in OCD

David L Pauls

Obsessive compulsive disorder (OCD) is a serious, potentially debilitating psychiatric condition affecting both children and adults.[1] Originally, OCD was considered to be rare in the general population.[2] However, recent data suggest that it is a common disorder with lifetime prevalence rates ranging from 1.9% to 3.3%.[3] This estimate was obtained from data collected using the Diagnostic Interview Schedule (DIS), a structured interview that elicited information to establish DSM-III diagnoses.[4] Furthermore, the lifetime prevalence rates of OCD in Canada, Puerto Rico, Germany, Taiwan, Korea and New Zealand were essentially the same as that reported in the USA. Rates ranged from 1.1% in Korea to 1.8% in New Zealand.

The influence of genetic factors has been suggested from the earliest descriptions of the disorder. Evidence for the influence of genetic factors has come from twin and family aggregation studies. Furthermore, drug treatment and functional neuroimaging studies have added strength to the genetic investigations by emphasizing the biochemical and biological nature of the disorder. In addition, recent molecular genetic studies suggest that specific genes may account for some of the variance in the manifestation of OCD.

Twin studies

Twin studies have provided evidence for the role of genetic factors in neuropsychiatric disorders.[5] The twin method consists of comparing the number of monozygotic (MZ) twins in which both members are affected (i.e. the pair is concordant) with the number of dizygotic (DZ) twin pairs concordant for the trait of interest. If the concordance of MZ twins is significantly higher than the concordance of DZ twins, it is taken as evidence for the contribution of genetic factors to the expression of the disorder under study. The similarity between twins can also be expressed as heritability. Heritability is defined as the proportion of phenotypic variance due to additive genetic factors. This statistic is descriptive but not predictive. A large heritability component does not preclude substantial influences by environmental factors within the population.[6,7] It does, however, serve as an indicator of a potentially significant biological etiology for a specific disorder.

In an early twin study of OCD completed in Japan, observed concordance rates were 80% among ten pairs of MZ twins and 50% among four pairs of DZ twins diagnosed as having 'obsessional neurosis'.[8] The small sample size precludes any definitive conclusions, but the data are consistent with a hypothesis of some genetic involvement.

In their review of the extant literature prior to 1986, Rasmussen and Tsuang found that 63% (32/51) of MZ twins were concordant for OCD.[9] When twins for whom zygosity was in doubt were eliminated from the sample, 65% (13/20) were concordant for OCD. These MZ concordance rates are similar to those reported for other affective and anxiety disorders (see reference 5 for review). However, the results need to be interpreted with caution because no data from DZ twins were available for comparison. Thus, it is not possible to determine the extent to which genetic factors contribute to the expression of OCD from these data.

Several twin studies not included in the Rasmussen and Tsuang review included data from DZ twins. Carey and Gottesman studied 15 MZ and 15 DZ twins ascertained from the Maudsley Twin Register.[10] These twins represented a consecutive series seen between 1910 and 1955. Each twin pair was personally interviewed using a structured interview documenting occurrence of psychiatric symptoms. This information was combined with hospital notes to determine the final psychiatric status. The investigators observed concordance rates of 87% and 47% for obsessive symptoms in MZ and DZ twins respectively.

In a study of 32 MZ and 53 DZ same-sex Norwegian twins, Torgersen investigated the concordance of anxiety disorders (including obsessive compulsive disorder).[11] The sample consisted of all twins born between 1910 and 1955 who were admitted for treatment of neurotic or borderline psychotic disorders at any time before 1977. Each twin was interviewed using a structured psychiatric interview which documented the lifetime occurrence of psychiatric symptoms. As in the Carey and Gottesman study, the interview data were combined with the hospital records to make DSM-III lifetime diagnoses. Six DSM-III anxiety disorders were examined: panic disorder, agoraphobia with and without panic, social phobia, obsessive compulsive disorder, and generalized anxiety disorder (GAD). No twins were concordant for the same DSM anxiety disorder. Thus, the author examined concordances in the larger context of an 'anxiety spectrum'. When the classification 'all anxiety disorders except GAD' was used to assigned affected status to the probands, the concordance rate was 45% in MZ pairs compared with 15% in DZ pairs ($p < 0.02$). This difference was not seen when considering GAD alone or for a proband diagnostic category of 'all anxiety disorders'. The author argued that these findings support the conclusion that genetic factors are important for the manifestation of non-GAD anxiety disorders. Thus, because OCD was included as part of the non-GAD anxiety disorder spectrum, genetic factors important in the etiology of OCD would have contributed to the finding of a higher MZ concordance.

Finally, Andrews et al administered structured psychiatric interviews to 186 MZ and 260 DZ twin pairs (446 pairs total) ascertained from the general Australian Twin Registry.[12,13] This study differs from those above in that ascertainment was not based on psychiatric index cases. Lifetime data for OCD, GAD, panic disorder, social phobia and major depressive disorder were obtained. Concordance rates for MZ and DZ twins were not significantly different for specific disorders. However, when the diagnoses were combined into a single category of 'neuroticism', the MZ concordances were significantly higher than those for the DZ twins (0.58 and 0.44 in female and male MZ twins, respectively, and 0.31, 0.27 and 0.33 in female, male and opposite-sex DZ twins, respectively). The data also support the conclusion that genetic factors are important for the manifestation of anxiety disorders in general.

The twin studies described above relied on categorical diagnoses. In 1984, Clifford and colleagues completed genetic analyses on data collected from 419 unselected twin pairs who had been given the 42-item version of the Leyton Obsessional Inventory (LOI).[14] Multivariate genetic analyses yielded separate heritability estimates of 44% for obsessional traits (as defined by the 10-item trait scale of the LOI) and 47% for obsessional symptoms (as defined by the 32-item symptom scale). These results support the earlier findings that genetic factors are important for the expression of the specific symptoms necessary for a diagnosis of OCD. They also support the notion that genetic factors influence the development and expression of obsessive-compulsive personality traits. These results suggest that the genetic factors important for symptoms and traits are in part independent from each other.

In summary, these twin studies provide some support for the hypothesis that genetic factors play a role in the manifestation of OCD. However, it is not clear whether these factors are specific for OCD or whether OCD is part of a broader, heritable anxiety spectrum. None of these studies provides conclusive evidence, but rather each serves as an indicator of a potentially significant genetic component in the etiology of OCD.

Family studies

A number of family studies on OCD and obsessional neurosis have been reported over a period of six decades. Overall, the data demonstrate that OCD is familial. Familial aggregation of a disorder is a necessary consequence if it is genetically transmitted. On the other hand, demonstration of familial aggregation is not sufficient to infer that there is genetic transmission. The family is the essential unit for transmitting not only genes but also the environmental and cultural factors that influence human behavioral phenotypes. These factors can have a large influence on phenotypic development and outcome. An understanding of these influences is crucial to the investigation of traits that typically have complex causes. Thus, while genetics alone may not explain familial aggregation of a disorder, demonstrating aggregation is an important step in understanding whether genetic factors are important.

Family study paradigms consist of:

- ascertainment of index cases (probands) affected with the disorder under investigation[15,16]
- estimation of the prevalence of the disorder among the biological relatives of probands
- comparison of rates of illness in families with those seen in control groups or in the general population.

The selection of an appropriate control group is essential. Control groups may be ascertained as relatives of unaffected cases, or as relatives of individuals affected with an unrelated disorder, or as relatives of randomly selected individuals from the general population. Population prevalence provides an alternative comparison, provided that the data were collected using similar (preferably identical) assessment instruments. Unfortunately, in most instances this kind of population information is not available, hence family-based control studies are necessary to obtain an appropriate comparison to determine whether a condition does run in families.

Two methods are used in determining the prevalence in relatives: the family history method, and the direct interview or family study method. Both methods endeavor to collect accurate symptom information on relatives that will allow the assignment of a best-estimate diagnosis.[17] The family history method relies on a single informant (usually the proband or the parent of a proband) to report diagnostic information on all first-degree relatives. In contrast, the direct interview method relies on personal assessment of all first-degree relatives to obtain diagnostic information. Because subjects sometimes fail to report symptoms in a direct interview (as may be the case in OCD, where sufferers tend to be secretive about their symptoms), the family history method can provide information that would be unavailable by direct interview alone. On the other hand, single informants may be unaware of specific symptoms in their first-degree relatives, in which case the prevalence in first-degree relatives may be underestimated; in this case, a direct interview offers an opportunity to gather otherwise unattainable information. To overcome the possible shortcomings of each method, both family history and direct interview data should be combined to assign diagnoses.

Family history method

All family aggregation studies completed prior to 1980 relied on the family history method. It is noteworthy that even using this method, the earliest studies demonstrated that obsessive compulsive illness was familial. Lewis reported that out of 306 first-degree relatives of obsessive compulsive patients, 37 parents and 63 siblings displayed pronounced obsessional traits, yielding a rate of 32.7%.[18] Brown found obsessional neuroses in 3 out of 40 parents and 4 of 56 siblings of obsessive compulsive neurotics; a rate of 7.3% among first-degree relatives.[19] Furthermore, Kringlen reported that 50% of the parents of 91 obsessional patients were 'nervous'.[20] Eighteen of the parents were diagnosed as obsessional neurotics. In 1967, Rosenberg reported a study of 547 first-degree relatives of 144 obsessional neurotics.[21] He reported an increased rate of psychiatric illness among first-degree relatives of obsessional neurotics, but there was no significant increase of obsessive compulsive disorder among those relatives. It is noteworthy that Rosenberg required that a relative be hospitalized in order to be included as affected. Similarly, Insel et al found no OCD among parents of 27 individuals with OCD;[22] however, when 20 parents were administered the Leyton Obsessional Inventory, 3 were found to have obsessive thoughts about contamination that were not recognized as problematic by their offspring proband. No information on siblings was provided. In 1986, Rasmussen and Tsuang described a sample of 44 patients who met DSM-III criteria for OCD.[9] Four of the 88 (4.5%) parents met the full criteria for OCD, and another 10 (11.4%) had significant obsessive compulsive traits that were not egodystonic. Combining the two groups into one obsessional category, 15.9% of the parents of OCD patients were affected.

Direct interview method

McKeon and Murray used a modified strategy to study first-degree relatives of 50 obsessive compulsive patients and those of matched controls.[23] These investigators requested that all relatives complete the LOI, and those who had high scores were interviewed directly. Although these relatives had a significantly higher rate of mental illness, there was only one who met criteria for obsessive compulsive neurosis. Thus, these investigators did not find any evidence to suggest that OCD was familial. One possible shortcoming of this study is the fact that individuals can have fairly low scores on the LOI by virtue of having only a few obsessions or compulsions, but those obsessions and compulsions can cause significant distress. Thus, it is possible that some affected relatives may have been missed in the ascertainment scheme employed.

Eight more recent studies of OCD directly interviewed all available relatives and used standard diagnostic criteria.[24–31] Findings from these studies provide further support for the hypothesis that there is a familial component important for the expression of some forms of OCD. Three of the studies focused on families of children with OCD,[24–26] whereas the other five reported data from families of adult probands.[27–31]

Lenane and colleagues studied 145 first-degree relatives of 46 children and adolescents with severe primary OCD who were consecutive admissions to a National Institute of Mental Health (NIMH) study of severe primary childhood OCD.[24] All parents and relatives were personally interviewed with structured psychiatric interviews. All diagnoses were based on DSM-III criteria. Seventeen per cent of the parents met criteria for OCD. No control group was examined.

Lenane and colleagues also examined the relationship between the probands' primary OCD symptoms and those of their respective relatives. They found no consistent pattern between parents and children, nor between older and younger siblings. Hence, a simple modeling hypothesis whereby OC symptoms are observed and learned by susceptible younger relatives was not supported by the data.[24]

A second study of childhood OCD interviewed the parents of 21 clinically referred children and adolescents with obsessive compulsive disorder.[25] Four of 42 (9.5%) parents received a DSM-III diagnosis of OCD. No information concerning rates of diagnosis in siblings was given. Interviewers and raters were not blind to the status of the proband and no control group was examined.

Finally, a third study examined 171 first-degree relatives of 54 childhood probands who were part of a drug treatment trial at NIMH.[26] Forty-six of these probands and their families had been studied previously by Lenane et al.[24] The later study was a 2-year to 7-year follow-up evaluation of those probands and their families. All diagnoses were made using DSM-III-R criteria. Thirteen per cent of all first-degree relatives met criteria for OCD.

Bellodi et al studied the families of 92 adult patients with OCD.[27] These patients were consecutive admissions for primary OCD at a specialty anxiety disorders clinic in Milan. All first-degree relatives were evaluated by either direct interview or family history. The rate of OCD among parents and siblings was only 3.4%. Although this rate was considerably lower than other published studies, it nevertheless represented a fourfold increase over population prevalence estimates for the Italian population. Furthermore, when probands were separated on the basis of age at onset (with 'early onset' defined as occurring at or up to 14 years of age), the frequency of OCD was significantly higher among the relatives of early-onset probands. The morbid risk for OCD among relatives of the 21 early-onset probands was 8.8% compared with 3.4% among the relatives of 71 later-onset probands. The number of relatives in each proband onset category was not given. As in previous studies, this group of investigators did not ascertain or assess a comparison sample.

Nicolini et al studied the families of 27 OCD probands ascertained through the Mexican Institute of Psychiatry in Mexico City.[28] Probands and all available first- and second-degree relatives were evaluated by direct interview, and unavailable relatives were evaluated by the family history method. All diagnoses were made with DSM-III-R criteria. A total of 268 first-degree relatives and 187 second-degree relatives were evaluated. Thirteen first-degree relatives received an OCD diagnosis, for a frequency of 4.9%; this was significantly different at the $p < 0.05$ level from the population prevalence of 1.8% in the USA.[3] The validity of this comparison rests on the assumption that the prevalence of OCD is similar in Mexico and the USA. The cross-national study suggests that this assumption is plausible, but it has not been confirmed.

A significant methodologic weakness of the five family studies just described was the lack of an appropriate comparison sample. Thus, it is not possible to determine whether the frequency of OCD observed among the family members in these studies was significantly higher than would be observed by these same investigators employing the same diagnostic methods in an independent sample of comparison subjects. Although the frequency of OCD in the families of affected probands could be compared with the population prevalence, the epidemiological investigations conducted to estimate that prevalence should have been done in the same geographic regions using identical assessment methods to ensure that the samples were comparable.

In contrast to these five studies, three more recent studies did include control groups. Black et al reported the findings from a study of 120 first-degree relatives of 32 OCD probands and 129 relatives of 33 psychiatrically normal controls.[29] Assessment of relatives was through direct structured interviews. Furthermore, the interviewer was blind to the proband's diagnostic status. All diagnoses were made using DSM-III criteria. The age-corrected morbid risk of OCD was 2.5% among relatives of OCD probands compared with 2.3% in relatives of controls; both values agree with the Epidemiology Catchment Area lifetime prevalence for OCD and thus provide no evidence that OCD is familial. However, the risk of a more broadly defined OCD was increased among the parents of OCD probands (15.6%) when compared with parents of normal individuals (2.9%).

A possible shortcoming of the Black study is that the investigators used only direct interview data to determine affected status. That is, they did not use all available information to assign diagnoses. In most family studies, the best estimate diagnostic process is used to assign the diagnosis to all probands and relatives.[17] This procedure includes direct interview information as well as family history data collected from multiple informants in the family. As noted above, individuals with OCD can be quite secretive about their symptoms, and in a direct interview might deny OC symptomatology, particularly if they had never sought help for their symptoms. It is noteworthy that Black and colleagues recorded that a number of family members were reported to have OC symptomatology by their relatives. Thus, if the direct interview and family history data had both been used to obtain diagnoses, it is likely that the recurrence risk for OCD among first-degree relatives would have been higher than among control relatives.

In a second controlled study 100 OCD probands, their 466 biological first-degree relatives and 113 comparison subjects were examined.[30] The 113 control group members were first-degree relatives of 33 psychiatrically unaffected subjects. All available first-degree relatives were interviewed directly and family history data were collected for all first-degree relatives from the interviewed participants. Best estimate diagnoses were assigned according to DSM-III-R criteria using all available clinical data. The frequency of OCD was significantly increased among relatives of OCD probands (10.3%) compared with control subjects (1.9%, $p < 0.005$).

Finally, Nestadt and colleagues studied 343 first-degree relatives of 80 OCD probands and 300 first-degree relatives of 73 control subjects.[31] Subjects were interviewed directly by clinicians using structured interviews. Additionally, a knowledgeable informant was interviewed about each subject. Consensus DSM-IV diagnoses were made using all available clinical data. Significant odds ratios were found for all definitions of the affected phenotype, indicating that first-degree relatives of cases met criteria for OCD-related phenotypes more often than first-degree relatives of controls. The actual risks to relatives were almost identical to the results reported by Pauls et al.[30] In general, using a more stringent criterion for affection status resulted in a more significant odds ratio. Interestingly, a stronger familial risk was found for obsessions than for compulsions.

It should be noted that in the Nestadt study as well as that of Pauls and colleagues, approximately half of the probands did not have any other relative with OCD; that is, they were isolated cases in their families. This pattern of familiality has also been observed in three other studies.[28,32,33] Thus, OCD appears to be a heterogeneous condition. Some cases are familial and others appear to have no family history of either OCD or other related conditions.

These studies of OCD probands and their relatives cumulatively provide strong evidence that some forms of OCD are familial. Taken together, the family and twin data reviewed here provide strong evidence that genetic factors play an important role in the manifestation of some forms of OCD.

Segregation analyses

Once familial aggregation of a disorder is established, a logical next step is to determine if the patterns of aggregation can be explained by Mendelian genetic models. Segregation analysis accomplishes this by examining the goodness-of-fit of genetic and non-genetic models to the observed data, and rejecting the models that do not explain the data well. Although segregation studies cannot prove the existence of genes, if the analyses reveal that the patterns within families are consistent with simple modes of inheritance, the results can be taken as evidence for the importance of genes in the etiology of the disorder. Three segregation analysis studies of nuclear families ascertained through a proband with OCD have been reported.

Nicolini and colleagues performed segregation analyses on data collected from 24 OCD families ascertained through the UCLA Child Psychiatry Clinic.[34] Eleven of the 24 probands had a positive family history of OCD. All available first-degree relatives were directly interviewed, with family history information used for unavailable relatives. Segregation analyses were performed including all affected individuals with a diagnosis of OCD, chronic motor tics, or Tourette's disorder. These investigators were unable to statistically reject either an autosomal dominant or autosomal recessive model.

More recent segregation analyses of a sample of 107 Italian families also provide evidence for genetic transmission of OCD.[35] Using regressive logistic models to test for possible models of genetic transmission, the authors determined that an autosomal dominant genetic model provided the best explanation for the pattern of transmission of OCD in these families. However, while the most parsimonious results suggested a single autosomal locus, other major gene solutions could also adequately explain the observed familial patterns.

Finally, Alsobrook et al reported the results of complex segregation analyses of 100 families ascertained through 100 adults with OCD.[36] Complex segregation analyses were completed using the computer program POINTER.[37] Using the entire data set and including as affected those relatives with a diagnosis of OCD, only the model of no transmission could be rejected. However, the polygenic model was nearly rejected. The lack of definitive results with the total sample could be due to the fact that, as noted above, approximately half of the families in this sample did not have any relatives affected with OCD.

Given these findings, these investigators undertook segregation analyses of the subset of families in which there were at least two individuals affected with DSM-III-R OCD. A total of 52 families were included in these analyses. Only relatives with OCD were included as affected. After correcting for the additional ascertainment bias introduced by selecting only familial cases of OCD, the models of no transmission, polygenic inheritance and single locus inheritance were all rejected. The best explanation of the patterns of transmission in these families was a genetic model that included genes of major effect as well as a polygenic background (the 'mixed model' of inheritance).

The results of all segregation analyses demonstrate that the transmission of OCD in families is difficult to model. This is not surprising given the clinical heterogeneity observed and the variability of family patterns that is evident from the several family studies published. However, in families in which the disorder is clearly familial (i.e. families in which there are at least two individuals with OCD), the results suggest a less complex mode of inheritance. The pattern in these families is consistent with a mixed model of transmission. The mixed model specifies a gene of major effect on a multigenic background. Thus, it is possible that there are several genes that influence components of OCD. Investigation of these factors in families with at least two affected individuals will allow a better evaluation of the underlying genetic and biological factors that might be important.

Candidate gene studies

Pharmacological and neurobiological studies have implicated several central neurotransmitter systems in the pathophysiology of OCD and related conditions. The strongest pharmacological evidence concerns the serotonergic system and the well-established efficacy of potent serotonin reuptake inhibitors in the treatment of OCD.[38,39] However, other systems have also been implicated. Specifically, central dopaminergic and opioid systems seem to be important in the expression of some forms of OCD.[39–42] More recently, several studies have implicated two closely related neuropeptides, arginine vasopressin (AVP) and oxytocin (OT) in the pathobiology of some forms of OCD.[43–46] Both AVP and OT have been implicated in the manifestation of memory, grooming, and sexual and aggressive behaviors.[47]

Given the apparent involvement of the serotonin and dopamine systems in OCD, a number of studies have examined several different genetic loci as possible candidate genes important for the manifestation of OCD. Genes examined include those coding for the serotonin transporter, the 5-HT_{2A}, 5HT_{2C}, DRD2, DRD3 and DRD4 receptors and the COMT locus. The results have been mixed, with some studies suggesting an association with OCD and others failing to replicate the findings.

The most recent family-based association study examined the association between OCD and the $5\text{-HT}_{1D\beta}$ autoreceptor gene.[59] This receptor is particularly interesting in OCD, as studies have shown that the $5\text{-HT}_{1D\beta}$ selective ligand sumatriptan may improve symptoms in OCD patients resistant to conventional pharmacotherapy.[60] Results of a transmission disequilibrium test showed a preferential transmission of the G allele of the G861C polymorphism of the $5\text{-HT}_{1D\beta}$ locus to OCD affected subjects ($z = 1.524$, $p < 0.01$).[61,62] As with the previous results, these findings need to be replicated on larger samples. If confirmed, the $5\text{-HT}_{1D\beta}$ receptor gene will be implicated in either the pathogenesis of OCD, or in the mechanism of the pharmacological response.

Given the complexity of the OCD phenotype, it is unlikely that any of these genes would have a major effect on the manifestation of the disorder. Given that current therapeutic agents appear to have their major influence on the serotonin and dopaminergic systems, it is possible that some of these genes might be important for effective treatment, but that does not necessarily imply that those same genes are involved in the etiology of OCD.

Future work

Because many published reports of genetic analyses suggest that some forms of OCD have a genetic basis, genetic linkage studies are warranted as the next step in our understanding of the inheritance of the disorder. Genetic linkage studies provide a powerful method for confirming the hypotheses of genetic involvement, because linkage results can demonstrate the existence of a genetic locus and help clarify the pattern of inheritance. The localization of genes responsible for the expression of OCD will be a major step forward in our understanding of the genetic and biological risk factors important for the expression of this disorder. In addition, this work will potentially allow the identification of non-genetic factors associated with the manifestation or the amelioration of the symptoms of the disorder.[63] On one hand, the identification of a linked marker will permit the design of more incisive studies to illuminate the biochemical basis of OCD by examination of the gene product and its impact on the manifestation of the disorder. On the other hand, by controlling for genetic factors it will be possible to document more carefully the non-genetic factors important for the expression of obsessions and compulsions. The ability to make use of genetic linkage and other aspects of genetic studies to design and carry out a study of non-genetic etiologic factors of a psychiatric illness is a significant methodological advancement that has not been possible heretofore.

Acknowledgements

This work was supported in part by grants NS-16648, MH-49351 and MH-00508 (an NIMH Research Scientist Award to Dr Pauls).

References

1   Calvocoressi L, Libman D, Vegso SJ et al, Global functioning of inpatients with obsessive-compulsive disorder, schizophrenia, and major depression, *Psychiatr Serv* (1998) **49**:379–81.

2   American Psychiatric Association Committee on Nomenclature and Statistics, *Diagnostic and Statistical Manual of Mental Disorders*, 3rd edn (American Psychiatric Association: Washington, DC, 1980).

3   Karno M, Golding JM, Sorenson SB, Burnam MA, The epidemiology of obsessive-compulsive disorder in five U.S. communities, *Arch Gen Psychiatry* (1988) **45**: 1084–99.

4   Robins LN, Helzer JE, Croughan J, Ratcliff KS, National Institute of Mental Health Diagnostic Interview Schedule: its history, characteristics, and validity, *Arch Gen Psychiatry* (1981) **38**:381–9.

5   National Institute of Mental Health's Genetics Workgroup, *Genetics and Mental Disorders* (National Institute of Mental Health, Washington, DC, 1998) 1–82.

6   Vogel F, Motulsky AG, *Human Genetics*, 2nd edn (Springer: New York, 1986).

7   Lewontin R, Comment on an erroneous conception of the meaning of heritability, *Behav Genet* (1976) **6**:373–4.

8   Inouye E, Similar and dissimilar manifestations of obsessive-compulsive neurosis in monozygotic twins, *Am J Psychiatry* (1965) **121**:1171–5.

9   Rasmussen SA, Tsuang MT, Clinical characteristics and family history in DSM-III obsessive-compulsive disorder, *Am J Psychiatry* (1986) **143**:317–22.

10   Carey G, Gottesman II, Twin and family studies of anxiety, phobic and obsessive disorders. In Klien DF, Rabkin J, eds, *Anxiety: New Research and Changing Concepts* (Raven Press: New York, 1981) 117–36.

11   Torgersen S, Genetic factors in anxiety disorder, *Arch Gen Psychiatry* (1983) **40**:1085–9.

12   Andrews G, Stewart G, Allen R, Henderson AS, The genetics of six neurotic disorders: a twin study, *J Affect Disord* (1990) **19**: 23–9.

13   Andrews G, Stewart G, Morris-Yates A, Holt P, Henderson AS, Evidence for a general neurotic syndrome, *Br J Psychiatry* (1990) **157**:6–12.

14   Clifford CA, Murray RM, Fulker DW, Genetic and environmental influences on obsessional traits and symptoms, *Psychol Med* (1984) **14**:791–800.

15   Khoury MJ, Beaty TH, Cohen BH, *Fundamentals of Genetic Epidemiology*. Monographs in Epidemiology and Biostatistics, vol. 19 (Oxford University Press: New York, 1993).

16   Weissman MM, Merikangas KR, John K, Wickramaratne P, Prusoff BA, Kidd KK, Family-genetic studies of psychiatric disorders, *Arch Gen Psychiatry* (1986) **43**: 1104–16.

17   Leckman JF, Sholomskas D, Thompson WD, Belanger A, Weissman MM, Best estimate of lifetime psychiatric diagnosis: a methodologic study, *Arch Gen Psychiatry* (1982) **39**:879–83.

18   Lewis A, Problems of obsessional illness, *Proc Roy Soc Med* (1935) **29**:325–36.

19   Brown FW, Heredity in the psychoneuroses, *Proc Roy Soc Med* (1942) **35**:785–90.

20 Kringlen E, Obsessional neurotics: a long term follow-up, *Br J Psychiatry* (1965) **111**:709–22.

21 Rosenberg CM, Familial aspects of obsessional neurosis, *Br J Psychiatry* (1967) **113**:405–13.

22 Insel T, Hoover C, Murphy DL, Parents of patients with obsessive compulsive disorder, *Psychol Med* (1983) **13**:807–11.

23 McKeon P, Murray R, Familial aspects of obsessive-compulsive neurosis, *Br J Psychiatry* (1987) **151**:528–34.

24 Lenane MC, Swedo SE, Leonard H, Pauls DL, Sceery W, Rapoport J, Psychiatric disorders in first degree relatives of children and adolescents with obsessive-compulsive disorder, *J Am Acad Child Adolesc Psych* (1990) **29**:407–12.

25 Riddle MA, Scahill L, King R et al, Obsessive compulsive disorder in children and adolescents: phenomenology and family history, *J Am Acad Child Adolesc Psych* (1990) **29**:766–72.

26 Leonard HL, Lenane MC, Swedo SE, Rettew DC, Gershon ES, Rapoport JL, Tics and Tourette's disorder: A 2- to 7-year follow-up of 54 obsessive-compulsive children, *Am J Psychiatry* (1992) **149**:1244–51.

27. Bellodi L, Sciuto G, Diaferia G, Ronchi P, Smeraldi E, Psychiatric disorders in the families of patients with obsessive-compulsive disorder, *Psychiatr Res* (1992) **42**:111–20.

28 Nicolini H, Weissbecker K, Mejia JM, Sanchez de Carmona M, Family study of obsessive-compulsive disorder in a Mexican population, *Arch Med Res* (1993) **24**(2):193–8.

29 Black DW, Noyes R, Goldstein RB, Blum N, A family study of obsessive-compulsive disorder, *Arch Gen Psychiatry* (1992) **49**:362–8.

30 Pauls DL, Alsobrook JP, Goodman W, Rasmussen S, Leckman JF, A family study of obsessive compulsive disorder, *Am J Psychiatry* (1995) **152**:76–84.

31 Nestadt G, Samuels J, Riddle M et al, A family study of obsessive-compulsive disorder, *Arch Gen Psychiatry* (2000) **57**:358–63.

32 Eapen V, Robertson MM, Alsobrook JP, Pauls DL, Obsessive compulsive symptoms in Gilles de la Tourette's syndrome and obsessive compulsive disorder: differences by diagnosis and family history, *Am J Med Genet* (1997) **74**:432–8.

33 Cavallini MC, Pasquale L, Bellodi L, Smeraldi E, Complex segregation analysis for obsessive compulsive disorder and related disorders, *Am J Med Genet (Neuropsych Genet)* (1999) **88**:38–43.

34 Nicolini H, Hanna G, Baxter L, Schwartz J, Weissbecker K, Spence MA, Segregation analysis of obsessive compulsive and associated disorders. Preliminary results, *Urs Medic* (1991) **1**:25–8.

35 Cavallini MC, De Bella D, Pasquale L, Henin M, Bellodi L, 5HT2C CYS23/SER23 polymorphism is not associated with obsessive-compulsive disorder, *Psychiatr Res* (1998) **77**:97–104.

36 Alsobrook JP, Leckman JF, Goodman WK, Rasmussen SA, Pauls DL, Segregation analysis of obsessive-compulsive disorder using symptom-based factors, *Am J Med Genet (Neuropsych Genet)* (1999) **88**(6):669–75.

37 Lalouel JM, Rao DC, Morton NE, A unified model for complex segregation analysis. *Am J Hum Genet* (1983) **35**:816–26.

38 Zohar J, Insel TR, Obsessive-compulsive disorder: psychobiological approaches to diagnosis, treatment and pathophysiology, *Biol Psychiatry* (1987) **2**:667–87.

39 Goodman WK, Price LH, Delgado PL et al, Specificity of serotonin reuptake inhibitors in the treatment of obsessive-compulsive disorder, *Arch Gen Psychiatry* (1990) **47**:577–85.

40 Hanna GL, McCracken JT, Cantwell DP, Prolactin in childhood obsessive-compulsive disorder: clinical correlates and response to clomipramine, *J Am Acad Child Adolesc Psych* (1991) **30**:173–8.

41 McDougle CJ, Goodman WK, Leckman JF, Barr LC, Heninger GR, Price LH, The efficacy of fluvoxamine in obsessive compulsive disorder: effects of comorbid chronic tic disorder, *J Clin Psychopharmacol* (1993) **13**:354–8.

42 McDougle CJ, Goodman WK, Leckman JF, Lee NC, Heninger GR, Price LH, Haloperidol addition in fluvoxamine-refractory obsessive compulsive disorder: a double blind placebo-controlled study in patients with and without tics, *Arch Gen Psychiatry* (1994) **51**:302–8.

43 Altemus M, Pigott T, Kalogeras KT et al, Abnormalities in the regulation of vasopressin and corticotropin releasing factor secretion in obsessive-compulsive disorder, *Arch Gen Psychiatry* (1992) **49**:9–20.

44 De Boer JA, Westenberg HGM, Oxytocin in obsessive compulsive disorder, *Peptides* (1992) **13**:1083–5.

45 Leckman JF, Goodman WK, North WG et al, Elevated levels of CSF oxytocin in obsessive compulsive disorder: comparison with Tourette's syndrome and healthy controls, *Arch Gen Psychiatry* (1994) **51**:782–92.

46 Swedo SE, Leonard HL, Kruesi MJ et al, Cerebrospinal fluid neurochemistry in children and adolescents with obsessive-compulsive disorder, *Arch Gen Psychiatry* (1992) **49**:29–36.

47 Leckman JF, Goodman WK, North WG et al, The role of central oxytocin in obsessive compulsive disorder and related normal behavior, *Psychoneuroendocrinology* (1994) **19**:723–49.

48 McDougle CJ, Epperson CN, Price LH, Gelernter J, Evidence for linkage disequilibrium between serotonin transporter protein gene (SLC6A4) and obsessive compulsive disorder, *Molec Psych* (1998) **3**:270–3.

49 Billett EA, Richter MA, King N, Heils A, Lesch KP, Kennedy JL, Obsessive compulsive disorder, response to serotonin reuptake inhibitors and the serotonin transporter gene. *Molec Psych* (1997) **2**:403–6.

50 Altemus M, Murphy DL, Greenberg B, Lesch KP, Intact coding region of the serotonin transporter gene in obsessive-compulsive disorder, *Am J Med Genet (Neuropsych Genet)* (1996) **67**:409–11.

51 Enoch MA, Kaye WH, Rotondo A, Greenberg BD, Murphy DL, Goldman D, 5-HT2A promoter polymorphism – 1438G/A, anorexia nervosa, and obsessive-compulsive disorder, *Lancet* (1998) **351**:1785–6.

52 Nicolini H, Cruz C, Camarena B et al, DRD2, DRD3 and 5HT2A receptor gene polymorphisms in obsessive-compulsive disorder, *Molec Psych* (1996) **1**:461–5.

53 Cruz C, Camarena B, King N et al, Increased prevalence of the seven-repeat variant of the dopamine D4 receptor gene in patients with obsessive-compulsive disorder with tics, *Neurosci Lett* (1997) **231**:1–4.

54 Di Bella D, Catalano M, Cichon S, Nothen MM, Association study of a null mutation in the dopamine

D4 receptor gene in Italian patients with obsessive-compulsive disorder, bipolar mood disorder and schizophrenia, *Psychiatr Genet* (1996) **6**: 119–21.

55 Karayiorgou M, Altemus M, Galke BL et al, Genotype determining low catechol-*O*-methyltransferase activity as a risk factor for obsessive-compulsive disorder, *Proc Nat Acad* Sci USA (1997) **94**:4572–5.

56 Alsobrook JP, Zohar AH, LeBoyer M, Chabane N, Ebstein RP, Pauls DL, Association between the COMT locus and obsessive compulsive disorder in females but not males, *Am J Med Genet (Neuropsych Genet)* (2000) in press.

57 Novelli E, Nobile M, Diaferia G, Sciuto G, Catalano M, A molecular investigation suggests no relationship between obsessive-compulsive disorder and the dopamine D2 receptor, *Neuropsychobiology* (1994) **29**:61–3.

58 Catalano M, Sciuto G, Di Bella D, Novelli E, Nobile M, Bellodi L, Lack of association between obsessive-compulsive disorder and the dopamine D3 receptor gene: some preliminary considerations, *Am J Med Genet (Neuropsych Genet)* (1994) **54**:253–5.

59 Mundo E, Richter MA, Hood K, Sam F, Macciardi F, Kennedy JL, The TDT/sib-TDT procedure applied to the study of the 2HT1Dβ receptor gene and obsessive-compulsive disorder, *Am J Hum Genet* (1999) **65**(suppl.):A437 [abstract].

60 Stern L, Zohar J, Cohen R, Sasson Y, Treatment of severe, drug resistant obsessive compulsive disorder with the 5HT1D agonist sumatriptan, *Eur Neuropsychopharmacol* (1998) **8**:325–8.

61 Spielman RS, Ewens WJ, A sibship test for linkage in the presence of association: the sib transmission/disequilibrium test, *Am J Hum Genet* (1998) **62**: 450–8.

62 Lappalainen J, Dean M, Charbonneau L, Virkkunen M, Linnoila M, Goldman D, Mapping of the serotonin 5-HY1Dβ autoreceptor gene on chromosome 6 and direct analysis for sequence variants, *Am J Hum Genet* (1995) **60**:157–61.

63 Kidd KK, New genetic strategies for studying psychiatric disorders. In *Genetic Aspects of Human Behavior* (Eds. Sakai T, Tsuboi T.) Igaku-Shoin Ltd: (Tokyo, 1985) 325–46.

7
The neuroanatomy of OCD

James V Lucey

Obsessive compulsive disorder (OCD) has been classified as an anxiety disorder within a rubric that also includes panic disorder (with or without agoraphobia), generalized anxiety disorder (GAD), and post-traumatic stress disorder (PTSD).[1] However, OCD is increasingly recognized as a brain disorder.[2] This neuropsychiatric view of OCD is supported first by the clinical association of OCD with diseases of the cerebral cortex and the neostriatum, and second by functional imaging data reporting associations between OCD and activity in corticostriatal brain regions.

Neuropsychiatric features of OCD

Since its clinical description by Westphal in 1878,[3] OCD has been associated with movement disorders and neurological conditions. Modern biological psychiatrists have reiterated these observations.[4] Although most OCD patients do not have gross cerebral lesions,[5] discrete lesions of the basal ganglia are associated with obsessive compulsive phenomena.[6] Obsessive compulsive disorder may develop following head injury,[7] birth injury,[8] or temporal lobe epilepsy.[5] Furthermore, neurosurgical treatments such as subcaudate tractotomy (in which cortical connections to deep striatal structures are severed) are still effective in rare resistant cases.[9]

More subtle neurological dysfunction (indicated by abnormalities of fine motor coordination, involuntary movements, sensory dysfunction and visuospatial errors) may be seen in OCD.[10] Furthermore OCD patients with high scores on a soft-signs neurological investigation are found to have increased ventricular volumes on computerized tomography.[11]

Movement disorders with striatal involvement are associated with increased incidence of OCD symptoms.[12,13] Symptoms of OCD are more common in postencephalitic Parkinson's disease and Sydenham's chorea,[12,14] and the presence of chorea implies basal ganglia involvement.

Gilles de la Tourette's syndrome (GTS) is a chronic neuropsychiatric disorder of childhood onset characterized by motor and phonic tics that wax and wane in intensity. Nearly 70% of GTS patients have obsessive compulsive symptoms.[15,16] Obsessive compulsive disorder is prevalent in up to 23% of first-degree relatives of GTS probands.[15] In some OCD samples 6% meet criteria for GTS.[16] Tics are repetitive, involuntary motor actions prevalent in up to 38% of OCD patients.[16] In a study of 50 Irish OCD outpatients, GTS was rare (2%), but tics were common.[17]

Functional anatomy of OCD

Just how the mammalian brain mediates obsession, compulsion and fear-related behaviour is far from clear. The data suggest that both normal and abnormal fear-related behaviours involve deep brain structures as well as the cerebral cortex.[18] Among the relevant deep structures involved are the components of the limbic system, including the hypothalamus, septum, hippocampus, amygdala and the cingulum; other bodies such as the thalamus, locus coeruleus, median raphe nuclei and the dentate/interposital nuclei of the cerebellum.

In OCD, according to the hypothesis of Gray,[19] the septo-hippocampal system (SHS) becomes oversensitive and labels too many incoming stimuli as important. This leads to persistent searching for those stimuli, with resultant checking and ritualizing. The role of the amygdala in the mediation of emotional behaviour has been recognized for over half a century.[20] It is now known to have a central part in the mediation of anxiety and conditioned fear.[21] The amygdala in humans has been shown to be involved in varied aspects of fear conditioning,[22] emotional memory,[23] and recognition of vocal intonations or facial expressions.[24] Indeed, different types of conditioned behaviour may be mediated by separate nuclei within the amygdala.[25]

Bilateral hippocampal lesions in rats produce repetitive behaviours that invariably include excessiveness, retarded extinction of learned behaviour, and increased avoidance.[26] There have been numerous cases of OCD symptoms arising following the development of diabetes insipidus or encephalitis lethargica.[12] According to Pitman, the similarities between symptoms and behaviours in OCD and neurobehavioural findings in animals with limbic structure damage 'are too close to be ignored by any theory of OCD causation'.[26]

There is also evidence to suggest that the cingulum (cingulate lobe), which is a medial area of the brain just dorsal to the corpus callosum, might be involved in OCD. Grey-Walter proposed that overactivity of the cingulate region led to compulsive behaviour.[27] Some of the most convincing evidence of the role of the cingulum in OCD comes from the literature on psychosurgery.[2] Tippin and Henn reported five severely obsessional patients who improved (with full remission in one) after modified leucotomy in which the medial 2–3 cm of white matter coming through the anterior cingulate gyrus was severed.[28] The procedure is thought to be effective by disrupting the thalamofrontal tract.

The neostriatal hypothesis of OCD

The orbitofrontal cortex, ventral striatum, globus pallidus and thalamus are anatomically connected in a loop.[29] These regions are thought to comprise a neural network involved in switching patterns of behaviour.[30] In addition to their role in motor control and movement disorder, the structures of the neostriatum contribute to skeletomotor, oculomotor, cognitive and limbic processes.[29,31] The neostriatal hypothesis of OCD states that (orbitofrontal) corticostriatal overactivity underlies the disorder.[32] These regions are most consistently reported as showing altered activity in resting state functional imagining of OCD.[33]

Imaging of OCD

In a study regarded as a landmark in the understanding of anxiety disorders, Baxter et al compared regional cerebral metabolic rate (rCMR^{glucose}) measured using [^{18}F]fluorodeoxyglucose (18-FDG) positron emission tomography (PET) in 14 OCD patients and depressed and healthy controls.[34] This revealed a significant increase in absolute levels of rCMR^{glucose} in the OCD left orbitofrontal gyrus and bilateral caudate nucleus.[34] This same group replicated their findings in 10 OCD patients without substantial depressive comorbidity, showing elevated rCMR^{glucose} in the orbital gyri and the caudate bilaterally.[35] The orbitofrontal regional rCMR^{glucose} was elevated in these patients, in marked contrast to the reduced rCMR^{glucose} seen in the prefrontal cortex of patients with unipolar depression.[34] Similar results were reported in a study of 8 non-depressed OCD patients compared with 30 healthy volunteers, in which 18-FDG PET demonstrated increased normalized rCMR^{glucose} in the right and left orbitofrontal cortex. No caudate differences were seen in this study.[36] Increased rCMR^{glucose} in the left orbitofrontal, right sensorimotor and bilateral prefrontal and anterior cingulate cortex in OCD was again found on PET in 18 adults with childhood-onset OCD compared with matched adult controls. Once again, both absolute and normalized caudate differences failed to reach significance.[14]

Three bilateral cortical regions were hypermetabolic in a PET study using oxygen 15 in OCD patients with a syndrome of obsessional slowness: the orbitofrontal cortex, the premotor cortex and the midfrontal cortex.[37] This study also examined striatal dopaminergic function using

[^{18}F]6-fluorodopa on PET and found normal uptake in the caudate, putamen and medial frontal cortex.[37]

Only one study has found a reduction in frontal cortical rCMR^{glucose} in OCD. In this study by Martinot et al the control group had substantially higher rCMR^{glucose} values than did others.[38] The patients were older and had a longer duration of illness (mean of 18 years). Baxter et al acknowledged that his subjects' elevated orbitofrontal rCMR^{glucose} could be related to high levels of anxiety.[34]

In PET studies after treatment with the serotonin reuptake inhibitor (SRI) clomipramine hydrochloride, rCMR^{glucose} was significantly reduced in the orbital frontal cortex and left caudate nucleus. Significant reductions were confined to the left caudate nucleus.[39] Likewise, Swedo et al found a reduction in rCMR^{glucose} in orbitofrontal cortex bilaterally in 13 OCD patients after 1 year of successful SRI treatment.[40] In one European study significant improvement on SRI treatment was also associated with decreased metabolism in the cingulate cortex.[41]

After treatment rCMR^{glucose} in the head of the right caudate nucleus was significantly reduced in responders, regardless of whether pharmacological or psychological treatment was used.[42] Changes in OCD symptoms correlated significantly with reductions in caudate rCMR^{glucose} in medicated subjects.[42] In a further study from the same centre, Schwartz et al replicated and extended these findings for a group of OCD patients ($n = 18$) treated exclusively with psychological methods.[43] The behaviour treatment involved exposure, response prevention and cognitive restructuring. Responders had significant bilateral decreases in rCMR^{glucose}, which were greater than those of non-responders. The authors concluded that a corticostriato–thalamic brain system is implicated in the mediation of OCD symptoms.[43] It seems that alteration of striatal rCMR^{glucose} is intimately associated with symptomatic recovery in OCD regardless of whether the treatment is pharmacologically or psychologically mediated.

Structural imaging

It seems improbable that OCD functional imaging differences could exist in the absence of some structural differences.[2] Some studies using computerized tomography and magnetic resonance imaging (MRI) found OCD caudate nuclear volume was reduced.[44,45] Normal caudate volumetric studies are also reported.[11,46,47] One structural MRI study of OCD patients, in comparison with healthy controls, found significantly less total white matter and significantly greater total cortex and opercular volumes, which correlated significantly with OCD syndrome severity.[48]

Studies during behavioural challenge

To focus on the neural mechanisms of the disease process itself, a number of nuclear medicine researchers use challenge paradigms, capitalizing on the experience of OCD behaviour therapists and the adaptability of PET imaging. By exposing OCD patients to increasing amounts of anxiogenic stimulus, these researchers attempt to visualize the brain basis of obsessions and rituals. Zohar et al administered behavioural challenges to 10 OCD patients while measuring rCBF with xenon 133 inhalation on single photon emission tomography (SPET).[49] Each patient was studied under three conditions: relaxation, imaginal flooding (in fantasy) and in vivo (actual) exposure to the anxiogenic stimulus. Subjective anxiety, obsessive compulsive ratings and autonomic measures (heart rate, blood pressure) increased significantly, but respiratory rate and P_{CO_2} did not change across the three conditions. Temporal cortical rCBF increased slightly during imaginal flooding, but rCBF decreased markedly in other cortical regions during in vivo exposure, when anxiety was highest by subjective and peripheral autonomic measures. As Gur et al had earlier proposed,[50] intense anxiety was associated with decreased rather than increased cortical perfusion, and related states of anxiety (e.g. anticipatory and obsessional anxiety) appeared to be associated with opposite effects on rCBF.

A later challenge study attempted to delineate the mediating neuroanatomy of OCD using the short half-life tracer labelled carbon dioxide ($[^{15}O]CO_2$), for repeated PET determinations of rCBF in 8 OCD patients during resting and provoked (symptomatic) states.[51] There was a significant increase in relative rCBF during symptomatic states in the right caudate nucleus, the left anterior cingulate cortex, and the orbitofrontal cortex bilaterally. Increases in the thalamus approached but did not reach statistical significance. Using a similar paradigm, McGuire et al examined 4 OCD patients using ^{15}O-labelled H_2O PET; each patient was scanned 12 times during the same session.[30] Each scan was paired with brief exposure to a hierarchy of contaminants that elicited increasingly intense urges to ritualize. There was a significant relationship between symptom intensity and neural activity (rCBF) in the right inferior frontal gyrus, caudate nucleus, putamen, globus pallidus and thalamus, and also the left hippocampus and posterior cingulate gyrus. Negative correlations were also seen in the right superior prefrontal cortex and temporoparietal cortex. These authors hypothesized that in OCD rCBF increases occurred in the orbitofrontal cortex, the neostriatum, the globus pallidus and the thalamus, in response to the urge to perform compulsive rituals. Hippocampal and cingulate changes appeared to relate to the associated anxiety.[30]

Functional MRI (fMRI) images in controlled and provoked (symptomatic) conditions were studied in 10 OCD patients and 5 healthy controls. No healthy subject revealed any activation. In contrast, symptomatic OCD patients activated areas consistent with previous PET and SPET imaging studies: these included the orbitofrontal, lateral frontal, anterior temporal, anterior cingulate and insular cortex, as well as the caudate and lenticular nuclei and the amygdala.[52]

SPET imaging

Other OCD functional imaging research groups have examined rCBF as uptake of technetium 99m hexamethyl propylenamine oxime (^{99m}Tc-HMPAO) on single photon emission tomography as an index of regional neural activity. Machlin et al used this method to estimate rCBF in 10 OCD patients and 8 controls using a single rotating SPET system with a 16 mm resolution; they found increased medial frontal rCBF in OCD.[53] There was no increase in orbitofrontal rCBF and no correlation with symptoms. They limited their comments to cortical regions.[53] Six of these patients were seen following treatment with an SRI (fluoxetine 20 mg per day) and their symptom ratings were significantly reduced. Subsequent SPET scanning showed that OCD medial frontal and whole brain blood flow were significantly reduced following treatment.[54]

Basal ganglia hypoperfusion was first seen on ^{99m}Tc-HMPAO SPET in a preliminary study in Canada.[55] In this study 11 OCD patients were evaluated for distribution of radioactive tracer: 8 demonstrated asymmetric perfusion, 6 of whom showed left-sided hypoperfusion of the basal ganglia. The study was limited since the analysis was qualitative and uncontrolled. A more rigorous analysis of ^{99m}Tc-HMPAO SPET uptake was provided by Edmonstone et al.[56] This study used a multidetector brain-dedicated SPET system with a resolution of 7.5 mm to compare OCD patients with healthy and depressed controls. Significant bilateral decreases in uptake were confined to the striatum (caudate and putamen) in the OCD group, despite an apparently paradoxical positive correlation between blood flow and anxiety.[56]

Rubin et al examined [133]Xe rCBF and regional cerebral ^{99m}Tc-HMPAO uptake on SPET in 10 adult men with OCD and 10 matched controls. With the ^{133}Xe method they found no rCBF differences, although there was a significant positive relationship between measures of illness severity and ^{133}Xe CBF.[57] Compared with healthy controls OCD patients had significantly elevated ^{99m}Tc-HMPAO uptake (rCBF) bilaterally in the orbitofrontal and the dorsal parietal cortex as well as the left posterofrontal cortex. In the OCD patients ^{99m}Tc-HMPAO uptake was significantly reduced bilaterally in the caudate nucleus but not in the putamen or thalamus.[57] Further support for the involvement of the orbitofrontal cortex and the caudate nucleus in OCD was provided by Rubin et al when they reported using regional ^{133}Xe CBF and ^{99m}Tc-HMPAO SPET to examine rCBF in OCD before and during treatment.[58] Despite clomipramine treatment, significant bilateral reductions in OCD caudate [99mTc]-HMPAO uptake remained.[58]

The SPET method was used to examine [99mTc]-HMPAO uptake or regional cerebral blood flow in seven brain regions in 30 OCD patients compared with 30 healthy controls.[17] The rCBF was lower in the OCD group in the right superior frontal cortex, right inferior frontal cortex, right caudate and right thalamus. It was also lower in the left superior frontal, left lateral temporal and left parietal cortex. In addition there were significant differences in the right medial temporal cortex, left lateral temporal cortex and left parietal cortex. Illness severity, compulsivity and obsessionality all correlated with regional blood flow.

The most prominent and widespread correlation was between the Yale–Brown Obsessive Compulsive Scale (Y–BOCS, see Appendix 1 p. 183) compulsion scores and rCBF. Compulsions correlated with rCBF to the right superior frontal cortex, right inferior frontal cortex, left inferior frontal cortex, left lateral temporal cortex, right medial temporal cortex, right and left parietal cortex and medial frontal (cingulate) cortex, and right and left thalami. Thus SPET data provide regional support for the neostriatal hypothesis.[59] However, these data did not support the view that overactivity in this loop is necessarily involved. Indeed, consistent with other [99mTc]-HMPAO SPET studies, reduced uptake was found in the OCD striatum. In OCD, striatal uptake of [99mTc]-HMPAO is consistently reduced on SPET.[17,55–58] Moreover, the evidence did not conclusively point to a selective OCD pathology within the orbitofrontal corticostriate loop. Involvement of the medial frontal (cingulate region) was also evident. Multiple regression analysis confirmed that changes in right parietal rCBF had prominent correlation with obsessive-compulsivity.[17] This is consistent with previous SPET and PET studies showing reduced OCD right parietal blood flow during exposure to ritual-evoking stimuli.[30,49] The evidence suggests that a role for the cingulate and the parietal lobe should not be omitted from neuroanatomical models of OCD. Thus other regions connected by the limbic loop are also involved in experience intrinsic to OCD.[60]

Neuroanatomy: an overview

Patients with OCD have been studied using a variety of functional imaging technologies such as positron emission tomography, single photon emission tomography and functional magnetic resonance imaging. They have been examined at rest, in comparison with depressed and anxious and healthy controls, on exposure to anxiogenic stimuli, and after pharmacological or psychological treatment. These patients repeatedly display brain differences involving the orbitofrontal cortex, cingulate gyrus, parietal lobe, caudate nucleus and thalamus. Such findings are among the most consistent imaging data in psychological medicine.

References

1　World Health Organization, *The ICD-10 Classification of Mental and Behavioural Disorders: Clinical Description and Diagnostic Guidelines* (WHO: Geneva, 1992), 142–5.

2　McGuire PK, The brain in obsessive-compulsive disorder, *Neurol Neurosurg Psych* (1995) **59**:457–9.

3　Westphal C, Dwangforstellungen, *Arch Psych Nervenkr* (1878) **8**: 734–50.

4　Rapoport JL, Obsessive-compulsive disorder and basal ganglia dysfunction, *Psychol Med* (1990) **20**:465–9.

5　Kettl PA, Marks IM, Neurological factors in obsessive compulsive disorder; two case reports and a review of the disorder, *Br J Psychiatry* (1986) **149**:315–19.

6　Tonkonogy J, Barreira P, Obsessive-compulsive disorder and caudate-frontal lesion, *Neuropsych Neuropsychol Behav Neurol* (1989) **2**:203–9.

7　McKeon J, McGuffin P, Robinson R, Obsessive compulsive neurosis following head injury – a report of four cases, *Br J Psychiatry* (1984) **144**:190–2.

8　Capstick N, Seldrup J, Obsessional states: a study of the relationship between abnormalities occurring at birth and the subsequent development of obsessional symptoms, *Acta Psych Scand* (1977) **56**:427–31.

9　Chiocca EA, Martuza RL, Neurosurgical treatment of the obsessive-compulsive disorder. In: Jenike MA, Baer L, Minichiello WE et al, eds, *Obsessive-compulsive Disorders: Theory and Management* (Mosby Year Book: St Louis, 1990) 283–94.

10　Hollander E, Schiffman E, Cohen B et al, Neurological soft signs in obsessive compulsive disorder, *Arch Gen Psychiatry* (1991) **48**:278–9.

11　Stein DJ, Hollander E, Chan S et al, Computed tomography and soft signs in obsessive compulsive disorder, (1993) *Psychiatr Res Neuroimaging* (1993) **50**: 143–50.

12　Von Economo C (Newman KO trans.), *Encephalitis Lethargica: Its Sequelae and Treatment* (Oxford University Press: London, 1932).

13　Swedo SE, Leonard HL, Childhood movement disorders and obsessive compulsive disorder, *J Clin Psychiatry* (1994) **55**(3): S32–7.

14　Swedo SE, Shapiro MB, Grady Cl et al, Cerebral glucose metabolism in childhood onset obsessive compulsive disorder, *Arch Gen Psychiatry* (1989) **46**:518–23.

15　Pauls DL, Towbin KE, Leckman JF et al, Gilles de la Tourettes syndrome and obsessive compulsive disorder, *Arch Gen Psychiatry* (1986) **43**:1180–2.

16　Pitman RK, Green RC, Jenike MA, Mesulam MM, Clinical comparison to Tourette's disorder with obsessive-compulsive disorder, *Am J Psychiatry* (1987) **144**(9): 1166–71.

17　Lucey JV, Costa DC, Blanes T et al, Regional cerebral blood flow in obsessive compulsive disordered patients at rest: differential correlates with obsessive-compulsive and anxious-avoidant dimensions, *Br J Psychiatry* (1995) **167**:629–34.

18　Marks IM, Phobic and obsessive compulsive phenomena: classification, prevalence and relationship to other problems. In: *Fears, Phobias and Rituals: Panic Anxi-*

ety and their Disorders (OUP: Oxford, 1987) 281–90.

19 Gray JA, *The Neuropsychology of Anxiety: An Enquiry into the Function of the Septohippocampal System* (Oxford University Press: New York, 1982).

20 Kluver H, Bucy PC, Preliminary analysis of the temporal lobes in monkeys, *Arch Neurol Psych* (1939) **42**:979–1000.

21 Davis M, The role of the amygdala in fear and anxiety, *Ann Rev Neurosci* (1992) **15**:353–75.

22 Bechara A, Tranel D, Damasio H, Adolphs R, Rockland C, Damasio AR, Double dissociation of the conditioning and declarative knowledge relative to the amygdala and hippocampus in humans. *Science* (1995) **269**:1115–18.

23 Cahill L, Babinsky R, Markowitsch H, McGaugh JL, The amygdala and emotional memory, *Nature* (1995) **377**:295–6.

24 Adolphs R, Tranel D, Damasio H, Damasio A, Impaired recognition of emotion in facial expression following bilateral damage to the human amygdala, *Nature* (1994) **372**:669–72.

25 Killcross S, Robbins TW, Everitt BJ, Differential types of fear-conditioned behaviour mediated by separate nuclei within the amygdala, *Nature* (1997) **388**: 377–80.

26 Pitman RK, Neurological aetiology of obsessive compulsive disorders? *Am J Psychiatry* (1982) **139**:139–40.

27 Grey-Walter WG, Viewpoints of mental illness: neurophysiological aspects, *Semin Psychiatry* (1977) **14**:211–31.

28 Tippin J, Henn FA, Modified leukotomy in the treatment of intractable obsessional neurosis, *Am J Psychiatry* (1982) **139**: 1601–3.

29 Alexander GE, DeLong M, Strick P, Parallel organisation of functionally segregated circuits linking the basal ganglia and cortex, *Ann Rev Neurosci* (1986) **9**:357–81.

30 McGuire PK, Bench CJ, Frith CD, Marks IM, Frackowiak RSJ, Dolan RJ, Functional anatomy of obsessive compulsive phenomena, *Br J Psychiatry* (1994) **164**:459–68.

31 Alexander GE, Crutcher MD, DeLong MR, Basal ganglia–thalamocortical circuits: parallel substrates for motor, oculomotor, prefrontal and limbic functions. In: Uylings HBM, Van Eden CG, DeBruin JPC, Corner MA, Feenstra MGP, eds, *Progress in Brain Research* (Elsevier: Amsterdam, 1990): 119–46.

32 Cummings JL, Frontal subcortical circuits and human behaviour. Review, *Arch Neurol* (1993) **50**(8):873–8.

33 Schwartz JM, Neuroanatomical aspects of cognitive behavioural therapy responses in obsessive compulsive disorder, *Br J Psychiatry* (1998) suppl. **35**:38–44.

34 Baxter LR, Phelps ME, Mazziotta JC, Guze BH, Schwartz JM, Selin CE, Local cerebral glucose metabolic rates in obsessive-compulsive disorder: a comparison with unipolar depression and normal controls, *Arch Gen Psychiatry* (1987) **44**:211–18.

35 Baxter LR, Schwartz JM, Mazziota JC et al, Cerebral glucose metabolic rates in non-depressed obsessive compulsive disorder, *Am J Psychiatry* (1988) **145**: 1560–3.

36 Nordahl TE, Benkelfat C, Semple WE, Gross M, King AC, Cohen RM, Cerebral glucose metabolic rates in obsessive compulsive disorder, *Neuropsychopharmacology* (1989) **2**:23–8.

37 Sawle G, Hymas N, Lees A, Frakowiak R, Obsessional slow-

ness: functional studies with positron emission tomography, *Brain* (1991) **114**:2191–202.

38 Martinot JL, Allilaire JF, Mazoyer BM et al, Obsessive-compulsive disorder: a clinical, neuropsychological and positron emission study, *Acta Psych Scand* (1990) **82**:233–42.

39 Benkelfat C, Nordahl TE, Semple WE, Local cerebral glucose metabolic rates in obsessive-compulsive disorder: patients treated with clomipramine, *Arch Gen Psychiatry* (1990) **47**:840–8.

40 Swedo SE, Pietrini P, Leonard HL et al, Cerebral glucose metabolism in childhood onset obsessive compulsive disorder: revisualization after pharmacotherapy, *Arch Gen Psychiatry* (1992) **49**:690–4.

41 Perani D, Colombo C, Bressi S et al, [18F]FDG PET study in obsessive-compulsive disorder. A clinical/metabolic correlation study after treatment, *Br J Psychiatry* (1995) **166**(2):244–50.

42 Baxter LR, Schwartz JM, Bergman KS et al, Caudate glucose metabolic rate changes with both drug and behaviour therapy for obsessive-compulsive disorder. *Arch Gen Psychiatry* (1992) **49**:681–9.

43 Schwartz JM, Stoessel PW, Baxter LR, Martin KM, Phelps ME, Systematic changes in cerebral glucose metabolic rate after successful behaviour modification treatment of obsessive-compulsive disorder, *Arch Gen Psychiatry* (1996) **53**:109–13.

44 Luxenberg JS, Swedo SE, Flament MF, Friedland RP, Rapoport J, Rapoport SI, Neuroanatomical abnormalities in obsessive-compulsive disorder detected with quantitative x-ray computed tomography, *Am J Psychiatry* (1988) **145**:1089–93.

45 Robinson D, Wu H, Munne RA et al, Reduced caudate nucleus volume in obsessive-compulsive disorder, *Arch Gen Psychiatry* (1995) **52**:393–8.

46 Garber HJ, Ananth JV, Chiu LC, Griswold VJ, Oldendorf WH, Nuclear magnetic resonance imaging in obsessive compulsive disorder, *Am J Psychiatry* (1989) **146**:1001–5.

47 Aylward EH, Harris GJ, Hoehn-Saric R, Barta PE, Machlin SR, Pearlson GD, Normal caudate nucleus in obsessive-compulsive disorder assessed by quantitative neuroimaging, *Arch Gen Psychiatry* (1996) **53**:577–84.

48 Jenike MA, Breiter HC, Baer L et al, Cerebral structural abnormalities in obsessive compulsive disorder: a quantitative morphometric magnetic resonance imaging study, *Arch Gen Psychiatry* (1996) **53**:625–32.

49 Zohar J, Insel TR, Berman KF, Foa EB, Hill JL, Weinberger DR, Anxiety and cerebral blood flow during behavioural challenge. Dissociation of central from peripheral and subjective measures, *Arch Gen Psychiatry* (1989) **46**:505–10.

50 Gur RC, Gur RE, Resnick SM, Skolnick BE, Alavi A, Reivch M, The effect of anxiety on cortical cerebral blood flow and metabolism, *J Cerebr Blood Flow Metab* (1987) **7**:173–7.

51 Rauch SL, Jenike MA, Alpert NM et al, Regional cerebral blood flow measured during symptom provocation in obsessive-compulsive disorder using oxygen 15-labeled carbon dioxide and positron emission tomography, *Arch Gen Psychiatry* (1994) **51**(1):62–70.

52 Breiter HC, Rauch SL, Kwong KK et al, Functional magnetic resonance imaging of symptom provocation in obsessive compulsive disorder, *Arch Gen Psychiatry* (1996) **53**:595–606.

53 Machlin SR, Harris GJ, Pearlson GD et al, Elevated medial frontal cerebral blood flow in obsessive compulsive patients: a SPET study, *Am J Psychiatry* (1991) **148**:1240–2.

54 Hoehn-Saric R, Pearlson GD, Harris GJ, Machlin SR, Camargo EE, Effects of fluoxetine on regional cerebral blood flow in obsessive-compulsive patients. *Am J Psychiatry* (1991) **148**:1242–5.

55 Adams BL, Warneke LB, McEwan AJ, Fraser BA, Single photon emission computerised tomography in obsessive compulsive disorder: a preliminary study, *J Psych Neurosci* (1993) **18**(3): 109–12.

56 Edmonstone Y, Austin MP, Prentice N et al, Uptake of 99m-Tc-exametazime shown by photon emission computerised tomography in obsessive compulsive disorder compared with major depression and normal controls, *Acta Psych Scand* (1994) **90**: 298–303.

57 Rubin R, Villanueva-Meyer J, Ananth J, Trajmar PG, Mena I, Regional Xenon-133 cerebral blood flow and cerebral technetium 99m-HMPAO uptake in un-medicated patients with obsessive-compulsive disorder and matched normal controls, *Arch Gen Psychiatry* (1992) **49**: 695–702.

58 Rubin R, Ananth J, Villanueva-Meyer J, Trajmar PG, Mena I, Regional 133xenon cerebral blood flow and cerebral 99mTc-HMPAO uptake in patients with obsessive-compulsive disorder before and during treatment, *Biol Psychiatry* (1995) **38**:429–37.

59 Lucey JV, Costa DC, Busatto GF et al, Caudate regional cerebral blood flow in obsessive compulsive disorder and panic disorder, *Psychiatr Res Neuroimaging* (1997) **74**:25–33.

60 Heimer L, The olfactory cortex and the ventral striatum. In: Livingston KE, Hornykiewesz O, eds, *Limbic Mechanisms* (Plenum: New York, 1978) 95–7.

8
Integrated pathophysiology

Donatella Marazziti

Serotonin and OCD

For more than a decade, the serotonin (5-HT) hypothesis of obsessive compulsive disorder (OCD) constituted a frame of reference for approaching the biology and pathophysiology of this disease. The first observations were those related to the effectiveness of clomipramine (a tricyclic antidepressant which preferentially blocks 5-HT reuptake), compared with other tricyclics or placebo, subsequently confirmed by the superiority of selective serotonin reuptake inhibitors (SSRIs) such as fluoxetine, fluvoxamine, paroxetine, sertraline and citalopram.[1–4] Moreover, indications of 5-HT involvement came also from cerebrospinal fluid (CSF) studies of 5-hydroxyindoleacetic acid (5-HIAA) in OCD, which have shown that a positive response to clomipramine was associated with high CSF levels of 5-HIAA,[5,6] while low levels correlated negatively with response to clomipramine and positively with obsessive compulsive (OC) symptom severity.[7] Other supporting evidence derived from the exacerbations of OC symptoms with 5-HT agonists led to the hypothesis of hypersensitivity of postsynaptic 5-HT receptors in OCD, a hypothesis that is still considered valid.[8–10]

Platelet studies

The main target of clomipramine and SSRIs, the 5-HT transporter, has been investigated in OCD for its presence in blood platelets: in fact, the active uptake for 5-HT in these cells is similar to that present in the brain, as demonstrated by the cloning of the two structures.[11,12] For some years, [^{3}H]-imipramine (^{3}H-IMI), has been mainly used to label it.[13] However, pharmacological studies in this field have shown heterogeneity of IMI binding sites when desipramine is used to define 'specific' binding.[14] Desipramine-defined IMI binding appears to be constituted by two subpopulations: only that being a protein, 5-HT-sensitive and sodium-dependent would be present in serotonergic neurons and related to the

5-HT transporter.[15] Insel et al found no difference in either 5-HT uptake or ^{3}H-IMI binding between healthy controls and OC patients,[5] and Weizman et al and Marazziti et al observed normal 5-HT uptake coupled with a reduced number of ^{3}H-IMI binding sites.[16,17] Black et al replicated Insel et al's finding of no change in ^{3}H-IMI binding, except for a decrease in such binding sites in clomipramine-treated patients,[18] while other studies have shown a decreased number of ^{3}H-IMI binding sites and a decreased affinity for 5-HT uptake,[19] as well as an increased velocity of 5-HT uptake, with no change in ^{3}H-IMI binding.[20] Subsequently, it has been demonstrated that the more selective ligand [^{3}H]-paroxetine (^{3}H-Par) binds to a single site, probably corresponding to the neuronal transporter,[21,22] and a significant decrease in the number of ^{3}H-Par binding sites, as compared with healthy controls, has been more recently reported by two groups.[23,24] Such a decrease appears to constitute a state-dependent marker, as it is reversed by successful treatment with different SSRIs.[25] In addition, this and other reports suggest that the patients showing the most 'severe' serotonergic abnormalities are those who respond better to the drugs and, therefore, link the serotonergic alteration to a positive response to serotonergic drugs.[25–27]

Pharmacological responses

The identification of at least 17 subtypes of 5-HT receptor[28] has led to the question of which subtype or subsystem might be primarily implicated in OCD. Besides the blockade of the 5-HT transporter, clomipramine enhances the responsiveness of the postsynaptic 5-HT$_{1A}$ receptor and provokes a desensitization of 5-HT$_{2C}$ receptors, while SSRIs cause a decrease in somatodendritic and terminal autoreceptor responsiveness.[29] The net increase in 5-HT release provoked by the two actions is particularly evident in the orbitofrontal cortex, an area that appears primarily implicated in OCD, after an 8-week time lag consistent with the delayed response to these drugs typical of OCD patients and at variance with depression. In addition, high doses of SSRIs are required to elicit this effect, in agreement with the clinical observation that OCD patients need higher doses than depressed patients. The effect of 5-HT in the orbitofrontal cortex has been linked to 5-HT$_2$-like receptors, since it is reversed by prolonged administration of 5-HT$_2$ antagonists. Clinical observation supports the notion that drugs blocking the 5-HT transporter display antiobsessional properties by increasing serotonergic transmission: both metergoline and ritanserin, non-selective 5-HT antagonists, seem to provoke symptoms in drug-remitted patients.[30,31] The role of 5-HT$_2$-like receptors is supported by preliminary observations of the antiobsessional effect of psilocybin, a hallucinogen with 5-HT agonist properties,[32] and by the clinical benefit in resistant OCD of atypical neuroleptics, such as risperidone, with a 5-HT$_2$/D$_2$ profile.[33]

Drug challenge tests

Another useful approach for exploring receptor subtypes is represented by drug challenge tests. Although the related findings are questionable because no sufficiently selective compound is currently available, nevertheless these tests provide dynamic studies of the receptors and raise interesting suggestions. The most frequently employed challenge uses m-chlorophenylpiperazine (m-CPP),[8,9,34] a partial 5-HT agonist with 5-HT$_{1A}$, 5-HT$_{1B/D}$, 5-HT$_{2C}$, 5-HT$_2$ receptor agonist and 5-HT$_2$ receptor antagonist properties, which also inhibits 5-HT reuptake and displaces ^{3}H-Par binding to the 5-HT transporter, provoking exacerbation of OC symptoms. In contrast, 2-chloro-6(-1-piperazinyl)pyrazine (MK-212), a 5-HT$_{1A}$ and 5-HT$_{2C}$ receptor agonist, provokes no behavioural effect in OCD.[35] The main difference between m-CCP and MK-212 is represented by the fact that the latter compound shows no affinity for 5-HT$_{1B/D}$ receptors. The possible role of 5-HT$_{1B/D}$ receptors was investigated by means of sumatriptan, an agonist at this level, but data are still meagre and controversial: while some authors reported exacerbation of obsessive symptoms,[36] others did not observe any change in 15 patients except a significant increase in growth hormone response.[37] Certainly, the matter needs to be further investigated, perhaps with 5-HT$_{1B/D}$ receptor agonists with better brain-penetrating properties than sumatriptan, which does not easily pass the blood-brain barrier.

Receptor subtypes

The overall data suggest the involvement of the following 5-HT receptor subtypes: 5-HT$_{1A}$, 5-HT$_{2A}$, 5-HT$_{2C}$ and 5-HT$_{1B/D}$ receptors. The 5-HT$_{1A}$ receptor subtype does not appear to be altered in OCD patients, as shown by the absence of effect after challenge with ipsapirone, a 5-HT$_{1A}$ receptor agonist,[38] and by the lack of clinical efficacy of buspirone,[39] so that the use of this drug in augmentation strategies is no longer recommended. The question of the role of the 5-HT$_{2A}$, 5-HT$_{2C}$ and 5-HT$_{1B/D}$ receptors in OCD is still open and deserves further investigation. However, we cannot disregard the potential involvement of other receptor subtypes: in particular, the 5-HT$_{5A}$ and 5-HT$_6$ subtypes where clomipramine seems to interact, and 5-HT$_{1F}$ where sumatriptan displays agonistic activity to the same degree as that exerted at the level of 5-HT$_{1D}$ receptors. With regard to other receptor subtypes, the status of 5-HT$_3$ receptors was explored with ondansetron, a drug which displays a high affinity at this level, given to 11 OCD patients before intravenous administration of m-CPP.[40] The findings of this study, showing that m-CPP provoked exacerbation of OCD symptoms and that pretreatment with ondansetron did not change this response, seem to exclude the involvement of 5-HT$_3$ receptors in OCD, although further data – in particular comparisons with control groups – are needed.

Intracellular mechanisms

Since a receptor is just the first step of a subsequent cascade of events, from a biochemical point of view, much interest is focused on the intracellular regulation of the 5-HT transporter and receptors. Some reports have underlined a link between 5-HT reuptake and protein kinase of type C (PKC) which inhibits the process,[41] and type A, which enhances 5-HT reuptake.[42] Protein kinase C belongs to a class of phosphorylases present at high concentration in the brain.[43-45] Diacylglycerol, derived from the hydrolysis of phosphatidylinositol 4,5-bisphosphate (PIP$_2$), stimulates PKC by increasing its affinity for calcium and membrane phospholipids deriving from receptor-mediated hydrolysis and by promoting its translocation from the cytosol to the particulate fraction.[46-48] We investigated the effect of the activation of PKC on 5-HT reuptake in a group of patients with OCD compared with a control group, and observed that the velocity of the reuptake decreased significantly in both OCD patients and healthy controls, although to a greater degree in OCD patients. This decrease in V_{max} of OCD patients was significantly more robust than in healthy controls, indicating that the mechanism is 'more active' in OCD.[49] This phenomenon could perhaps be attributed either to hyperresponsiveness of the 5-HT reuptake system, or to hyperactivation of PKC in OCD. Such a latter condition might in turn reflect increased endogenous production of diacylglycerol as a result of a hyperactive phosphatidylinositol (PI) pathway. A stimulation of the PI pathway in OCD is congruent with data showing a worsening of OCD symptoms following administration of a 5-HT$_{2C}$ receptor agonist such as m-CPP,[8,9] a non-specific a 5-HT$_{2C}$ receptor agonist, and it is well known that 5-HT$_{2C}$ receptors are linked with a G protein activating phospholipase C.[50] However, other receptors are linked with phospholipase C, including 5-HT$_{2A}$, dopamine and muscarinic receptors: interestingly, atypical neuroleptics are agonistic at 5-HT$_{2A}$ receptor level. Hyperactivity of the PI pathway might provoke an alteration in the normal balance existing between the PI pathway and the cyclic AMP pathway, and increased PKA activity in OCD patients has been demonstrated.[51] There is also evidence of the therapeutic effect of inositol, a naturally occurring isomer of glucose that acts as a precursor in the PI pathway in OCD.[52] It can, therefore, be hypothesized that OCD may perhaps be due to an imbalance of the two main transduction pathways, cAMP and PI, with a prevalence of the second and a consequently higher activation of PKC, relative to PKA, given the cross-talk between the two main second messengers at the level of different effectors.

Besides the PI pathway, SSRIs and antidepressants have been shown to upregulate the cAMP–response element binding protein (CREB, a transcription factor) cascade, as well as the expression of the brain-derived neurotrophic factor (BDNF).[53] Interestingly, CREB is a substrate for both PKA and PKC, and 5-HT$_{2C}$ agonists seem to influence CREB and BDNF expression. Therefore, we strongly believe that the elucidation of these mechanisms will shed new light on disorders such as OCD, where SSRIs are effective.

Beyond 5-HT

Although the findings implicating 5-HT in the pathophysiology of OCD are increasing at a level and with a convergence that are not found in any other psychiatric disorder, the hypothesis that this disorder might be due to a unique neurochemical abnormality contrasts with the observation that at least 30% of patients do not respond to SSRIs.[1,54] In addition, it is plausible that the overall clinical heterogeneity of the patients might be supported by different biological mechanisms. Evidence has been accumulating of disturbances in other neurotransmitters, such as dopamine, noradrenaline (norepinephrine) and in some neuropeptides in the aetiology of OCD: however, in some cases, the findings are meagre and controversial. More agreement exists on the role of immune mechanisms in a subtype of childhood OCD.

Dopamine

Apart from 5-HT abnormalities, the most consistent findings described in OCD are those related to the dopamine system. The earliest data derived from the observation of increased stereotypic behaviours in animals undergoing manipulation of the dopamine system. Subjects with disorders of the basal ganglia (a dopamine area), such as Gilles de la Tourette's syndrome, postencephalitic Parkinson's or tic syndrome disorder, often present with OC symptoms. Cocaine users also suffer from stereotypic and OC behaviours. These observations have led to the use of dopamine blockade by typical and atypical neuroleptics as augmentation strategies in refractory OCD.[55]

Direct evaluation of peripheral dopamine markers is still very difficult. We demonstrated an increased activity of platelet sulfotransferase, an enzyme involved in the catabolism of dopamine, in a group of drug-free OCD patients, which can reflect an increased level of circulating neurotransmitter.[17]

Noradrenaline

Several studies have reported abnormalities in the noradrenaline system, based mainly on the positive response of OCD patients to the α_2-adrenergic agonist clonidine.[9,56,57] However, evaluation of the role of the noradrenaline system in OCD by means of challenge tests has been controversial.

An interesting study showed lower CSF concentrations of tyramine and homovanileic acid in 44 OCD patients than in normal controls or in patients with Tourette's syndrome (who also exhibited increased levels of noradrenaline).[58] However, CSF findings, as well as those deriving from plasma or urine measurements, should be considered with caution given the low reliability and sensitivity of the methods used.

Neuropeptides

New interest has been directed towards two related neuropeptides, arginine vasopressin and oxytocin, as increased levels have been reported in patients with pure OCD.[59] It has been proposed that the oxytocin system is involved in the regulation of affiliative behaviours and parental bonding, and that a disturbance at this level may be related to the pathophysiology of a specific OCD subtype. Altemus et al showed that clomipramine increased CSF oxytocin levels in children and adolescents with OCD.[60]

Another neuropeptide reported to be more abundant in the CSF of OCD patients is somatostatin;[61] in experimental animals this produces behaviours resembling compulsive acts.[62]

Opioid peptides

Amongst other activities, the opioid system is involved in the regulation of conditioned responses, and it has therefore been hypothesized that it might have a role in the onset and maintenance of OCD symptoms. A few clinical observations have suggested the possible usefulness of tramadol, a major analgesic, in refractory OCD patients.[63,64]

Immunological alterations in OCD

There is broad agreement that some forms of childhood OCD may be due to immunological alterations, on the basis of the possible shared involvement of basal ganglia abnormalities in OCD and Sydenham's chorea, both resulting from infection-driven autoimmune processes.[65] Sydenham's chorea is a manifestation of rheumatic fever, following an infection provoked by group A β-haemolytic streptococci, which is thought to derive from the production of antibodies cross-reacting with neurons of the basal ganglia.[66] The relationship between OCD and Sydenham's chorea is strengthened by clinical observations showing that more than 80% of children with the latter condition show obsessions and compulsions both before and concomitantly with, choreic movements,[67] and that one-third of OCD children present with choreiform movements.[68] As a result, the hypothesis has emerged that infections with group A β-haemolytic streptococci might produce conditions grouped together under the acronym PANDAS (Paediatric Autoimmune Neuropsychiatric Disorders Associated with Streptococci), including subtypes of paediatric OCD and tics.[69,70] However, the observation has been made that even viral infections might trigger the autoimmune process leading to OCD.[71,72] Furthermore, patients with rheumatic fever show a high level of antineural antibodies against the caudate nucleus,[73] and a particular antigen in B lymphocytes reacting with a monoclonal antibody, D8/D17.[74,75] Such an antigen has been shown to be stable in different populations and over time; more interestingly, it is also present in patients with childhood OCD, Tourette's syndrome and chronic tic disorder.[76] Preliminary data also indicate its presence in subjects with autism.[77] Although the relationship between the antigen identified by the D8/17 antibody and the pathophysiology of the various disorders is not yet clear, it has been considered either to be an immunological marker of susceptibility to rheumatic fever,[75] or to be linked to the motor component of the various disturbances.[78]

The literature regarding immunological factors in adult OCD is sparse. Cytokine production appears to be normal in OCD patients, at variance with depressed patients.[79] Barber et al evaluated T-lymphocyte subsets in chronic OCD patients in the acute phase, but were unable to find any difference in comparison with healthy controls, either before or after successful clomipramine treatment.[80] On the other hand, the possible involvement of the immune system in some subtypes of OCD is supported by the finding of a relationship between the severity of the disorder and interleukin-6 (IL-6) and IL-6 receptor levels[81] and by the observation of decreased concentrations of plasma cytokines, such as interleukin-1β and tumour necrosis factor-α,[82] related to hyperactivity of the noradrenergic system and of the hypothalamus–pituitary–adrenal (HPA) axis. Increased levels of cells carrying the CD8$^+$ antigen and decreased levels of those carrying – i.e. suppressor and helper lymphocytes, respectively, have been demonstrated in adult OCD patients.[83] The role of immune factors in OCD is also supported by the report of increased CSF levels of immunoglobulin G antibodies against herpes virus type 1 suggestive of a chronic infection, in a sample of adult patients,[72] but the specificity of these findings needs to be clarified.

All these observations are intriguing, but much research remains to be done. In particular, it would be helpful to identify familial, clinical or symptomatological features that might be linked to immunological disturbances. The presence of such disturbances suggests the use of non-conventional treatments, in particular antibiotics or immunomodulators;[67,71] however, the results of the first pilot study of penicillin prophylaxis in children with PANDAS were negative.[84]

Conclusion

Considerable advances have been made in the understanding of the pathogenesis of OCD. A wealth of evidence in favour of abnormalities of the 5-HT system has, however, led to the notion that 'the best is yet to come'.[85] That is, if the role of 5-HT is undoubted, there are a number of open questions related to the serotonergic system still to be answered. Are the serotonergic disturbances primary or secondary? Are they involved in the pathophysiological chain or only in the phamacological response? In addition, the serotonergic abnormalities found in OCD have been reported also in other psychiatric conditions and therefore cannot be considered nosologically specific, but rather linked to a dimension (or dimensions) cutting across different diagnostic entities. Although much research is still required, some authors have already highlighted relationships between the 5-HT transporter and personality traits,[86] aggressive features,[87] anxiety traits,[88] and the overvalued ideation typical of the early, romantic phase of a love relationship.[89] In addition, if the successful use of SSRIs has highlighted the key role of the 5-HT transporter, latest developments in the mode of action of these drugs suggest the involvement of different 5-HT receptor subtypes yet to be identified and, probably, of second messengers. Taken together, these findings suggest further possibilities in the treatment of OCD through the modulation of new therapeutic targets. Thus, compounds acting on specific 5-HT receptor subtypes, such as the 5-HT_{2A}, 5-HT_{2C}, 5-HT_{5A} receptors and probably others, or compounds that inhibit PKC, potentiate PKA or act on various G-protein subunits, seem to represent potential antiobsessive drugs.

The role of other neurotransmitters has not been deeply explored, mainly because of the lack of sensitive and reliable research tools; nevertheless, the role of noradrenaline, dopamine and some peptides deserves further investigation.

Disturbances of the immune system continue to be reported in some OCD subtypes – particularly in the childhood form, although data also indicate immune dysregulations in adult OCD. Immunological alterations appear to be different in children and in adults, probably reflecting different pathophysiological mechanisms such as autoimmune and possibly primary processes in children, and perhaps secondary alterations in adulthood. The immunological disturbances may be also related to specific dimensions, as a correlation between the antigen D8/17 and repetitive behaviours in autistic subjects has been reported.[77]

In conclusion, the availability of research data from a number of sources has served to underline the complexities of OCD, which appears to be heterogeneous not only clinically but also in terms of its pathophysiological mechanisms. Probably there exist multiple causes with the ability to trigger OCD symptoms according to individual vulnerability (genetically based?) or exposure to certain agents (infections?), with prevalence varying at different ages. The involvement of various neuro-transmitters/neuroreceptors and circuitries and the balance between them might provide an explanation of the presence of more or less obsessions or compulsions or both, or of one type of obsession or compulsion over another.

Alternatively, the neurochemical imbalance may produce disturbances in dimensions yet to be identified that might explain the overlapping of symptoms and the common drug response observed in various psychiatric conditions. Without doubt, the identification of these common dimensions that constitute the 'core' feature of the disorder, will constitute an intriguing area for future research.

References

1 Montgomery SA, Pharmacological treatment of obsessive-compulsive disorder. In: Hollander E, Zohar J, Marazziti D, Olivier B, eds, *Current Insights in Obsessive-compulsive Disorder* (John Wiley: Chichester, 1994) 215–26.

2 Piccinelli M, Pini S, Bellantuono C, Wilkinson C, Efficacy of drug treatment in obsessive-compulsive disorder, *Br J Psychiatry* (1995) **166**:424–43.

3 Greist JH, Jefferson JW, Kobak KH et al, Efficacy and tolerability of serotonin transport inhibitors in obsessive-compulsive disorder, *Arch Gen Psychiatry* (1995) **52**:53–60.

4 Fineberg N, Refining treatment approaches in obsessive-compulsive disorder, *J Clin Psychopharmacol* (1996) **11**:(suppl. 5) 13–22.

5 Insel TR, Mueller EA, Alterman I et al, Obsessive-compulsive disorder and serotonin: is there a connection? *Biol Psychiatry* (1985) **20**:1174–88.

6 Thoren P, Asberg M, Cronholm B, Clomipramine treatment of obsessive-compulsive disorder: a controlled clinical trial, *Arch Gen Psychiatry* (1980) **37**:1281–9.

7 Asberg M, Thoren P, Bertilsson L, Clomipramine treatment of obsessive disorder: biochemical and clinical aspects, *Psychopharmacol Bull* (1981) **18**:13–21.

8 Zohar J, Insel TR, Obsessive-compulsive disorder: psychobiological approaches to diagnosis, treatment and pathophysiology, *Biol Psychiatry* (1987) **22**:667–87.

9 Hollander E, Fay M, Cohen B et al, Serotonergic and noradrenergic sensitivity in obsessive-compulsive disorder: behavioral findings, *Arch Gen Psychiatry* (1988) **145**:1015–23.

10 Zohar J, Insel TR, Zohar-Kadouch RC, Hill J, Murphy DL, Serotonergic responsivity in obsessive-compulsive disorder. Effect of chronic clomipramine treatment, *Arch Gen Psychiatry* (1988) **45**:167–72.

11 Lesch KP, Wolozin BL, Murphy DL, Riederer P, Primary structure of the human platelet serotonin uptake: identity with the brain serotonin transporter, *J Neurochem* (1993) **60**:2319–22.

12 Rausch JJ, Hutchinson J, Li X, Correlations of drug action between human platelets and human brain 5HT, *Biol Psychiatry* (1995) **137**(suppl.):600.

13 Meyerson LR, Ieni JR, Wennogle LP, Allosteric interaction between

the site labelled by ^{3}H-imipramine and the serotonin transporter in human platelets, *J Neurochem* (1987) **48**:560–5.

14 Hrdina PD, Differences between sodium-dependent and desipramine-defined ^{3}H-imipramine binding in intact human platelets, *Biol Psychiatry* (1989) **25**:576–84.

15 Marcusson JO, Fowler CJ, Hall H et al, 'Specific' binding of ^{3}H-imipramine to protease-sensitive and protease-resistant sites, *J Neurochem* (1985) **44**:705–11.

16 Weizman R, Carmi M, Hermesh H et al, High-affinity imipramine binding and serotonin uptake in platelets of eight adolescent and ten adult obsessive-compulsive patients, *Am J Psychiatry* (1986) **143**:335–9.

17 Marazziti D, Hollander E, Lensi P et al, Peripheral markers of serotonin and dopamine function in obsessive-compulsive disorder, *Psychiatry Res* (1992) **42**:41–51.

18 Black DW, Kelly M, Myers C, Noyes R, Tritiated imipramine binding in obsessive-compulsive volunteers and psychiatrically normal controls, *Biol Psychiatry* (1990) **27**:319–27.

19 Bastani B, Arora RC, Meltzer HY, Serotonin uptake and imipramine binding in the blood platelets of obsessive-compulsive disorder patients, *Biol Psychiatry* (1991) **30**:131–9.

20 Vitiello B, Shimon H, Behar D et al, Platelet imipramine binding and serotonin uptake in obsessive-compulsive patients, *Acta Psychiatr Scand* (1991) **84**:29–32.

21 Mann CD, Hrdina PPD, Sodium dependence of ^{3}H-paroxetine binding and 5-^{3}H-hydroxytryptamine uptake in rat diencephalon, *J Neurochem* (1992) **59**:1856–61.

22 Mellerup ET, Plenge P, Engelstoft M, High-affinity binding of ^{3}H-paroxetine and ^{3}H-imipramine to human platelet membranes, *Eur J Pharmacol* (1983) **96**:303–9.

23 Marazziti D, Rossi A, Gemignani, G et al, Decreased ^{3}H-paroxetine binding in obsessive-compulsive patients, *Neuropsychobiology* (1996) **34**:184–7.

24 Sallee FR, Richman H, Beach K et al, Platelet serotonin transporter in children and adolescents with obsessive-compulsive disorder or Tourette's syndrome, *J Am Acad Child Adolesc Psych* (1996) **35**: 1647–56.

25 Hollander E, DeCaria C, Wong CM, Aronowitz B, Predictors of SSRI treatment response in OCD and autism. Paper presented at the XXI CNP Congress, Glasgow, 12–16 July 1998, abstract 191.

26 Zohar Y, Sasson Y, Chopra M, Groos R, Predictors of response in OCD. Paper presented at the XXI CNP Congress, Glasgow, 12–16 July 1998, abstract 191.

27 Marazziti D, Predictors of response, *Eur Neuropsychopharmacol* (1997) **27**(suppl. 2): 101–2.

28 Hoyer D, Martin G, 5-HT receptor classification and nomenclature: towards a harmonization with the human genome, *Neuropharmacology* (1997) **36**:419–28.

29 Blier P, De Montigny C, Possible serotonergic mechanisms underlying the antidepressant and anti-obsessive-compulsive disorder responses, *Biol Psychiatry* (1998) **44**:312–23.

30 Benkefalt C, Murphy DL, Zohar J et al, Clomipramine in obsessive-compulsive disorder: further evidence for a serotonergic mechanism of action, *Arch Gen Psychiatry* (1989) **46**:23–8.

31 Erzegovesi S, Ronchi P, Smeraldi E, 5-HT2 receptor and fluvoxamine in obsessive-compulsive disorder, *Hum Psychopharmacol* (1992) **7**:287–9.

32 Moreno FA, Delgado PL, Hallucinogen-induced relief of obsessions and compulsions, *Am J Psychiatry* (1997) **145**:1037–8.

33 McDougle CJ, Update on pharmacologic management of OCD: agents and augmentation, *J Clin Psychiatry* (1997) **58**(suppl 12): 11–17.

34 Pigott TA, Zohar J, Hill JL et al, Metergoline blocks the behavioral and neuroendocrine effects of orally administered m-chlorophenylpiperazine in patients with obsessive-compulsive disorder, *Biol Psychiatry* (1991) **29**:418–26.

35 Bastani B, Nash F, Meltzer H, Prolactin and cortisol response to MK-212, a serotonin agonist, in obsessive-compulsive disorder, *Arch Gen Psychiatry* (1990) **47**:946–51.

36 Stern L, Zohar J, Hendler T et al, The potential role of 5-HT$_{1D}$ receptors in the pathophysiology of obsessive-compulsive disorder. *CNS Spectrum* (1998) **3**(8):46–9

37 Ho Pian KL, Westenberg HGM, van Megen HJGM, Den Boer JA, Sumatriptan (5-HT$_{1D}$ receptor agonist) does not exacerbate symptoms in obsessive-compulsive disorder, *Psychopharmacology* (1998) **140**:365–70.

38 Lesch KP, Hoh A, Disselkamp-Tietze J et al, 5-Hydroxytryptamine$_{1A}$ receptor activity in obsessive-compulsive disorder: comparison of patients and controls, *Arch Gen Psychiatry* (1991) **48**:540–7.

39 McDougle CJ, Goodman WK, Leckman JF et al, Limited therapeutic efficacy of addition of buspirone in fluvoxamine-refractory obsessive-compulsive disorder, *Am J Psychiatry* (1993) **150**: 647–9.

40 Broock A, Pigott TA, Hill JL et al, Acute intravenous administration of ondansetron and m-CPP, alone and in combination, in patients with obsessive-compulsive disorder (OCD): behavioral and biological results, *Psychiatr Res* (1998) **79**:11–20.

41 Anderson G, Horne WC, Activators of protein kinase C decrease serotonin transport in human platelets, *Biochim Biophys Acta* (1992) **1137**:331–7.

42 De Vivo M, Maayani S, Inhibition of forskolin stimulation adenylate cyclase activity by 5-HT receptor agonist, *Eur J Pharmacol* (1985) **119**(3):231–4

43 Nishizuka Y, Studies and perspective of protein kinase C, *Science* (1986) **233**:305–12.

44 Kikkawa U, Kishimoto A, Nishizuka Y, The protein kinase C family: heterogeneity and its implications, *Ann Rev Biochem* (1989) **58**:31–44.

45 Wilkinson SE, Hallam TJ, Protein kinase C: is pivotal role in cellular activation over-stated? *TIPS* (1994) **15**:53–7.

46 Berridge MJ, Downes CP, Hanley MR, Lithium amplifies agonist-dependent phosphatidylinositol responses in brain and salivary glands, *Biochem J* (1982) **206**:587–95.

47 Ashendel CL, The phorbol ester receptor: a phospholipid-regulated protein kinase, *Biochim Biophys Acta* (1985) **822**:219–42.

48 Weiss S, Ellis J, Hendley DD, Lenox RH, Translocation and activation of protein kinase C in striatal neurons in primary culture: relationship to phorbol dibutyrate actions on the inositol phosphate generating system and neurotransmitter release, *J Neurochem* (1989) **52**:530–6.

49 Marazziti D, Rossi A, Masala I et al, Regulation of the platelet serotonin transporter by protein

kinase C in the young and elderly, *Biol Psychiatry* (1999) **45**:443–7.

50 Wang HY, Friedman E, Central 5-Hydroxytryptamine receptor-linked protein kinase C translocation: a postfunctional postsynaptic signal transduction system, *Mol Pharmacol* (1989) **37**:75–9.

51 Perez J, Tardito D, Ravizza L, Racagni G, Mori S, Maina G, Altered cAMP-dependent protein kinase in platelets of patients with obsessive-compulsive disorder, *Am J Psychiatry* (2000) **157**:284–6.

52 Fux M, Levine J, Aviv A, Belmaker RH, Inositol treatment of obsessive-compulsive disorder, *Am J Psychiatry* (1996) **153**:1219–21.

53 Duman RS, Novel therapeutic approaches beyond the serotonin receptor, *Biol Psychiatry* (1998) **44**:324–35.

54 Sasson Y, Zohar Y, New developments in obsessive-compulsive disorder research: implications for clinical management, *J Clin Psychopharmacol* (1996) **11**(suppl. 5): 3–12.

55 McDougle J, Goodman WK, Price LK et al, Neuroleptic addition in fluvoxamine-refractory obsessive-compulsive disorder, *Am J Psychiatry* (1990) **150**:647–9.

56 Knesevich JW, Successful treatment of obsessive-compulsive disorder with clonidine hydrochloride, *Am J Psychiatry* (1982) **139**:360–5.

57 Hollander E, De Caria C, Nitescu A et al, Noradrenergic function in obsessive-compulsive disorder: behavioral and neuroendocrine responses to clonidine and comparison to healthy controls, *Psychiatr Res* (1991) **37**:161–77.

58 Leckman JF, Goodman WK, Anderson GM et al, Cerebrospinal fluid biogenic amines in obsessive-compulsive disorder, Tourette's syndrome, and healthy controls, *Neuropsychopharmacology* (1995) **12**:73–86.

59 Leckman JF, Goodman WK, North WG et al, Elevated levels of CSF oxytocin in obsessive-compulsive disorder: Comparison with Tourette's syndrome and healthy controls, *Arch Gen Psychiatry* (1994) **51**:782–92.

60 Altemus M, Swedo SE, Leonard B et al, Changes in cerebrospinal fluid neurochemistry during treatment of obsessive-compulsive disorder with clomipramine, *Arch Gen Psychiatry* (1994) **51**:794–803.

61 Altemus M, Pigott T, L'Hereux F et al, Cerebrospinal fluid somatostatin in obsessive-compulsive disorder, *Am J Psychiatry* (1993) **15**:460–4.

62 Pitman RK, Animal models of compulsive behaviour, *Biol Psychiatry* (1989) **26**:189–98.

63 Shapira NA, Goldsmith TD, Keck PE, Open label study of tramadol hydrochloride in treatment-refractory obsessive-compulsive disorder, *Depress Anx* (1997) **6**:170–3.

64 Goldsmith TD, Shapira NA, Keck PE, Rapid remission of OCD with tramadol hydrochloride, *Am J Psychiatry* (1999) **156**:660–1.

65 Swedo SE, Sydenham's chorea: a model for autoimmune neuropsychiatric disorders, *JAMA* (1994) **272**:1788–91.

66 Bronze MS, Dale JB, Epitopes of streptococcal M proteins that evoke antibodies that cross-react with human brain, *J Immunol* (1993) **151**:2820–8.

67 Swedo SE, Leonard HL, Kiessling LS, Speculations on antineuronal antibody-mediated neuropsychiatric disorders of childhood, *Pediatrics* (1994) **93**:323–6.

68 Denckla MB, Rapoport JL, Neurological examination. In: Denckla MB, Rapoport JL, eds, *Obses-*

sive-compulsive Disorder in Children and Adolescents (American Psychiatric Press: Washington DC, 1989) 107–18.

69 Swedo SE, Leonard HL, Mittleman B et al, Identification of children with paediatric autoimmune neuropsychiatric disorders associated with streptococcal infections by a marker associated with rheumatic fever, *Am J Psychiatry* (1997) **154**:110–12.

70 Swedo SE, Leonard HL, Garvey M et al, Paediatric Autoimmune Neuropsychiatric Disorders associated with Streptococcal Infections (PANDAS): a clinical description of the first fifty cases, *Am J Psychiatry* (1998) **55**: 264–71.

71 Allen AJ, Leonard HL, Swedo SE, Case study: a new infection-triggered autoimmune subtype of pediatric OCD and Tourette's syndrome, *J Am Acad Child Adolesc Psych* (1995) **34**:307–11.

72 Khanna S, Ravi V, Shenoy PK et al, Cerebrospinal fluid viral antibodies in obsessive-compulsive disorder in an Indian population, *Biol Psychiatry* (1997) **41**: 883–90.

73 Husby G, van den Rijn I, Zabriskie JB et al, Antibodies reacting with cytoplasm of subthalamic and caudate nuclei neurons in chorea and acute rheumatic fever, *J Exp Med* (1976) **144**:1094–110.

74 Zabriskie JB, Rheumatic fever: a model for the pathological consequences of microbial-host mimicry, *J Clin Exp Rheumatol* (1986) **4**:65–73.

75 Gibofsky A, Khanna A, Suh E, Zabriskie JB, The genetics of rheumatic fever: relationship to streptococcal infection and autoimmune disease, *J Rheumatol* (1991) **18**(suppl. 30): 1–5.

76 Murphy TK, Goodman WK, Fudge

MW et al, B Lymphocyte antigen D8/17: a peripheral marker for childhood-onset obsessive-compulsive disorder and Tourette's syndrome? *Am J Psychiatry* (1997) 154: **3**:402–7.

77 Hollander E, DelGiudice G, Simon L et al, B lymphocyte D8/17 and repetitive behavior in autism, *Am J Psychiatry* (1999) **156**:317–20.

78 Kiessling LS, Marcotte AC, Culpepper L, Antineuronal antibodies in movement disorders, *Pediatrics* (1993) **92**:39–43.

79 Weizman R, Laor N, Barber Y et al, Cytokine production in obsessive-compulsive disorder, *Biol Psychiatry* (1996) **40**:908–12.

80 Barber Y, Toren P, Achiron A et al, T cell subsets in obsessive-compulsive disorder, *Neuropsychobiology* (1996) **34**:63–6.

81 Maes M, Meltzer HY, Bosnan E, Psychoimmune investigation in obsessive-compulsive disorder: assay of plasma transferrin, IL-β and IL-6 receptors, and IL-1β and IL-6 concentrations, *Neuropsychobiology* (1994) **30**:57–60.

82 Brambilla F, Perna G, Bellodi L et al, Plasma interleukin 1 beta and tumor necrosis factor concentrations in obsessive-compulsive disorder, *Biol Psychiatry* (1997) **42**:976–81.

83 Marazziti D, Presta S, Pfanner C et al, Immunological alterations in adult obsessive-compulsive disorder, *Biol Psychiatry* (1999) **46**: 810–14.

84 Garvey MA, Perlmutter SJ, Allen AJ et al, A pilot study of penicillin prophylaxis for neuropsychiatric exacerbation triggered by streptococcal infections, *Biol Psychiatry* (1999) **45**:1564–71.

85 Greden JF, Serotonin: how much we have learned! So much to discover, *Biol Psychiatry* (1998) **44**: 309–11.

86 Lesch KP, Benge D, Heils A et al,

Association of anxiety-related traits with a polymorphism in the serotonin transporter gene regulatory region, *Science* (1996); **274**:1527–31.

87 Mazzanti C, Lappalainen J, Long JC et al, Role of the serotonin transporter promoter polymorphism in anxiety-related traits, *Arch Gen Psychiatry* (1998) **55**:936–40.

88 Coccaro EF, Kavoussi RJ, Sheline YI et al, Impulsive aggression in personality disorder correlates with tritiated paroxetine binding in the platelets, *Arch Gen Psychiatry* (1996) **53**:531–6.

89 Marazziti D, Akiskal HS, Rossi A, Cassano GB, Alteration of the platelet serotonin transporter in romantic love, *Psychol Med* (1999) **29**:741–5.

9
Practical pharmacotherapy

Joseph Zohar and Naomi Fineberg

Before 1980, the prognosis for obsessive compulsive disorder (OCD) was poor. The discovery of effective drug therapies revolutionized the outlook for sufferers, and paved the way for research into the neurobiology of OCD. In this chapter we attempt to answer the key clinical questions concerning drug treatment of OCD as far as possible using evidence derived from randomized, controlled trials (Table 9.1).

The serotonin hypothesis

Intensive pharmacological investigation has demonstrated that OCD responds selectively to drugs that act as potent inhibitors of the synaptic reuptake of serotonin (serotonin reuptake inhibitors, SRIs) – that is, clomipramine and the selective SRIs (Table 9.2). Drugs lacking these properties, such as the standard tricyclic antidepressants amitriptyline, desipramine and nortriptyline, and the monoamine oxidase inhibitors clorgyline and phenelzine, have been shown to be ineffective in randomized, controlled trials.[1,2] Studies looking at benzodiazepines, lithium and electroconvulsive therapy have not produced positive findings (reviewed by Zohar et al).[3] Antipsychotics also appear ineffective on their own, although they may have a role as agents of augmentation in cases where the response to the SRI is incomplete (see Chapter 11) or when a combination of OCD and tic disorder is present.

Table 9.1 Practical questions for OCD pharmacotherapy.

- What kind of drug?
- What dose?
- What are the side effects?
- What about comorbidity?
- How long should treatment continue, and what happens if treatment is discontinued?

Table 9.2 The pharmacological specificity of OCD.

Effective as monotherapy
Potent SRIs such as clomipramine, fluvoxamine, fluoxetine, sertraline, paroxetine and citalopram

Potential as agents of augmentation in combination with SRIs
Conventional antipsychotics such as haloperidol[a]
Atypical antipsychotics such as risperidone,[b] olanzapine[c]
Pindolol[d]

Ineffective
Tricyclic antidepressants (apart from clomipramine)
Monoamine oxidase inhibitors
Lithium
Benzodiazepines
Buspirone
Electroconvulsive therapy

[a]Effective in OCD with comorbid tics.[4]
[b]Effective in the absence of comorbid tics.[5]
[c]Efficacy not yet established in controlled studies.
[d]Positive and negative findings from controlled studies.[6,7]

The selectivity of the pharmacological response distinguishes OCD from the other anxiety disorders and from depression in which both noradrenergic and serotonergic medications appear to be equally potent.

Although the pharmacological data indicate a role for serotonin in the pathophysiology of OCD, neurobiological research has failed to produce consistent findings. It appears increasingly unlikely that the illness results from a specific abnormality in serotonin neurotransmission, and there may well be a variety of different biochemical abnormalities underpinning the disorder.

If this is the case, why then are the SRIs uniquely effective? Serotonin is understood to play an important role in modulating stress. Instead of repairing a specific serotonergic lesion, it is possible that the SRIs work in OCD by enhancing fundamental neuropsychological defence systems, which rely on serotonin activity to function adequately.[8]

Clomipramine: the first effective drug for OCD

The discovery that clomipramine is an effective treatment for OCD was an important breakthrough. Clomipramine can be distinguished from the other tricyclic drugs by its more powerful SRI activity, although its effects are not exclusively serotonergic. The first reports of the successful treatment of OCD by clomipramine appeared as early as the 1960s.[9,10] The seminal study by Montgomery specifically excluded depressed individuals and demonstrated efficacy against placebo using a relatively modest fixed daily dose (75 mg) in a small, carefully selected group.[11] Later, larger studies confirmed that daily doses of up to 300 mg were effective in adults and children, both in the presence and absence of depression (reviewed by Zohar et al).[3] It is now established beyond doubt that the antiobsessional effect of clomipramine does not depend upon an anti-depressant effect.

Characteristics of the drug effect

Obsessive compulsive disorder shows a slow, gradual improvement which starts within a few days of the initiation of treatment and continues for months thereafter. These characteristics were demonstrated most clearly in the treatment-naive populations entering the early clomipramine studies. In large multicentre studies of clomipramine,[12] there was a 40–45% improvement measured by the Yale–Brown Obsessive Compulsive Scale (Y-BOCS, see Appendix 1, p. 183)[13] by the 10-week end-point. This represented a considerable functional improvement, involving substantial reductions in time spent on obsessions and compulsions.

Extension studies in OCD have shown that gains continue to be made for at least 2 years as long as treatment is continued, and patients need to be encouraged to persevere during the early stages when progress can seem frustratingly slow.

Selective SRIs

Efficacy compared with clomipramine

Convincing evidence from large-scale randomized, placebo-controlled studies supports the efficacy of fluvoxamine, fluoxetine, sertraline, paroxetine and citalopram in OCD (reviewed by Zohar et al).[3] The size of the treatment effect reported for the selective serotonin reuptake inhibitors (SSRIs) was smaller than that reported in the earlier trials of clomipramine – probably because the early studies included fewer treatment-resistant cases. Claims that clomipramine shows stronger efficacy (by, for example, Piccinelli et al)[14] have been challenged by the results from controlled comparator studies (Table 9.3). Many of these studies were underpowered,[25] but the trial by Bisserbe et al was large enough to show a significant advantage for sertraline over (low-dose) clomipramine,[23] and since the advantage was only for some efficacy measures and only in the intent-to-treat group, the superiority is not clear-cut. Even larger studies showed equivalent efficacy for clomipramine and paroxetine.[21,22]

Table 9.3 Comparing SSRIs with clomipramine: controlled studies.

Study	No.	Design	Outcome
Fluoxetine			
Piggott et al (1990)[15]	11	CMI vs FLX	CMI = FLX
Lopez-Ibor et al (1996)[16]	55	CMI vs FLX	CMI = FLX on primary criterion
			CMI > FLX on other criteria
Fluvoxamine			
Smeraldi et al (1992)[17]	10	CMI vs FLV	CMI = FLV
Freeman et al (1994)[18]	64	CMI vs FLV	CMI = FLV
Koran et al (1996)[19]	42	CMI vs FLV	CMI = FLV
	37		
Milanfranchi et al (1997)[20]	26	CMI vs FLV	CMI = FLV
Rouillon (1998)[21]	105	CMI vs FLV	CMI = FLV
	112		
Paroxetine			
Zohar and Judge (1996)[22]	99	CMI	CMI > Placebo
	201	vs PAR	PAR > Placebo
	99	vs Placebo	
Sertraline			
Bisserbe et al (1997)[23]	82	CMI	SER = CMI
	86	vs SER	
Citalopram			
Pidrman and Tuma (1998)[24]	24	CIT vs CMI	CIT = CMI

CIT, citalopram; CMI, clomipramine; FLV, fluvoxamine; FLX, fluoxetine; PAR, paroxetine; SER, sertraline.

SSRIs as first-line treatment for OCD

In the face of equivalent efficacy, the choice of SRI depends to a large extent on the side-effect profile of the compound. An important advantage of the SSRIs over clomipramine lies in their greater acceptability. The risk of dangerous side effects such as convulsions (occurring in up to 2% patients on clomipramine, 0.1–0.5% patients on higher-dose SSRIs), cardiotoxicity and cognitive impairment is substantially lower on SSRIs. Clomipramine shares the unpalatable side effects associated with the older tricyclics, including dry mouth, constipation, weight gain and blurred vision. The SSRIs are better tolerated, although they are responsible for more asthenia, insomnia and nausea. Whereas all SRIs are associated with impaired sexual performance, clomipramine (up to 80% of cases) is worse than the SSRIs (up to 30% of cases) in this respect. In the comparator studies, the drop-out rate for adverse effects on clomipramine (around 17%) was consistently higher than that for the SSRIs (around 9%). In fact, the greater tolerability of sertraline was thought to have explained its superior effect on the intent-to-treat analysis in the comparator study by Bisserbe et al (Table 9.3).[23]

Improved safety and tolerability and lower rates of premature discontinuation offer considerable benefits for long-term treatment, and indicate that the SSRIs should be considered the treatment of choice, with clomipramine reserved as a second-line treatment for those who cannot tolerate SSRIs or who have failed to respond to them.

Differences between SSRIs

Choosing between SSRIs is difficult because their effects are so similar. In the absence of comparator data, the selection of a drug largely depends upon personal preference. Occasionally the possibility of a drug interaction influences the choice. Sertraline and citalopram are relatively weak inhibitors of the hepatic cytochrome P450 enzymes which metabolize commonly prescribed drugs, and may be preferred if drug interactions are likely to be a problem. Fluoxetine and paroxetine are powerful inhibitors of the CYP 2D6 isoenzyme, which metabolizes tricyclic antidepressants, antipsychotics, antiarrhythmics and beta-blockers. Fluvoxamine inhibits both CYP 1A2, which eliminates warfarin and tricyclics, and CYP 3A4, which metabolizes benzodiazepines and some antiarrhythmics. Fluoxetine has a long half-life and an active metabolite resulting in fewer withdrawal effects, which can be advantageous for patients who forget to take their tablets.

Comorbid depression

Obsessive compulsive disorder is commonly complicated by comorbid depression, and roughly one-third of patients presenting for treatment are concurrently depressed. Comorbid OCD has received little investigation because most treatment studies have attempted to exclude depressed patients to keep the sample 'pure'. Moderate levels of depression do not appear to interfere with the antiobsessional response to SRI treatment.[22] Comorbid depression responds together with the OCD, sharing its characteristic selectivity for serotonergic antidepressants.[26]

Unlike drug treatment, studies looking at behaviour therapy have shown that moderately high levels of baseline depression adversely affect the outcome of treatment.[27] It has been suggested that this disadvantage may be neutralized by augmenting the behaviour therapy with an SSRI,[28] although the studies looking at this area have not been able to disentangle the antiobsessional effects of the medication from those of the behavioural intervention. These findings suggest that for depressed patients with OCD the first-line treatment should be with an SRI.

Dosage

What is the most effective dose for OCD?

In order to answer this question studies need to compare multiple fixed doses of the active drug, preferably also with placebo (Table 9.4).[29] Neither clomipramine nor fluvoxamine have been examined in this way, although the results from the study by Montgomery suggest that 75 mg clomipramine is the minimum effective dose.[11] Fixed-dose studies have been performed for paroxetine, fluoxetine, sertraline and citalopram. In the case of paroxetine, a positive dose–response relationship was clearly demonstrated; the 40 mg and 60 mg daily doses showed efficacy while the 20 mg dose did not differ from placebo.[33] The fluoxetine studies produced similar results: whereas all three fixed doses (20 mg, 40 mg, 60 mg) were effective, there was a trend toward greater improvement in the group receiving 60 mg a day, which became significant when data were pooled from more than one study centre.[31,35] There is another clear suggestion of a dose–response relationship for fluoxetine, with the 20 mg daily dose producing an effect no different from placebo, while the 40 mg and 60 mg doses produced the best effect.[30]

The results for sertraline are not clear. In a study that has been criticized for lack of statistical power, the 50 mg and 200 mg doses were superior to placebo, whereas the 100 mg dose was not.[32] In the preliminary report of a fixed-dose study, 20 mg of citalopram were found to be effective, with a suggestion of increasing effect over time with increasing dose.[34]

Table 9.4 Placebo-controlled fixed-dose studies in OCD.

Study	Fixed dose (mg)	N	Duration (weeks)	Positive dose–response relationship?
Fluoxetine				
Montgomery et al (1993)[30]	20/40/60	214	8	Yes[a]
Tollefson et al (1994)[31]	20/40/60	355	13	No
Sertraline				
Greist et al (1995)[32]	50/100/200	324	12	No
Paroxetine				
Wheadon et al (1993)[33]	20/40/60	348	12	Yes
Citalopram				
Montgomery (1998)[34]	20/40/60	352	12	Yes[b]

[a]Marginally significant benefit for medium and higher doses on primary analysis (total Y-BOCS, see Appendix 1, p. 183), $p = 0.059$; significant on 'responder' analysis ($p < 0.05$).

These results have been interpreted to suggest that the higher dose levels (e.g. 40–60 mg of fluoxetine, paroxetine or citalopram) are associated with better antiobsessional efficacy. Some experts use even higher doses, particularly in resistant cases, but in the absence of controlled data this practice cannot be recommended without reservation.

Dose titration: the key to effective pharmacotherapy

Improvements in OCD take several weeks to become established, irrespective of the dose, and it is helpful to warn patients about this from the outset. Gastrointestinal symptoms often occur in the first days of SSRI treatment and are usually short-lived; they can be ameliorated by starting at the lower dose levels and slowly titrating upwards, monitoring for longer-term side effects such as sleep disturbance and headache, which may become more prominent as the dose increases. Sexual function should be carefully monitored, and if necessary strategies such as medication to restore potency (e.g. sildenafil, mianserin, cyproheptadine,[36]) dose reduction or short 'drug holidays' can be considered if the patient is stable.

Sufferers from OCD are notoriously poor at recognizing their own improvements. Systematic use of observer-rated scales such as the Y-BOCS[13] (see Appendix 1, p. 183) and the assistance of reliable informants can be invaluable in the clinical setting.

Is treatment effective over the longer term?

Because OCD is a long-term illness, we need to be confident that the treatment effect endures. Evidence for long-term efficacy can be derived from a variety of sources. Some investigators have taken treatment responders from acute-phase studies and followed them on 'uncontrolled' SRI for up to 2 years, with the result that the response has increased over time without tolerance developing.[37] A study by Wagner et al demonstrated ongoing efficacy and tolerability for open-label sertraline, up to 1 year, in a large cohort of children and adolescents.[38]

The evidence from controlled studies is more convincing. Cottraux et al found that fluvoxamine continued to show superiority over placebo, in the face of concomitant behaviour therapy in both groups, after 6 months of double-blind treatment (Table 9.5).[39]

A small number of studies have followed treatment responders for up to 1 year under double-blind, placebo-controlled conditions, and have found that the treatment effect was sustained (Table 9.5). Patients continued to improve on active treatment, whereas those remaining on placebo did not. In the large extension study by Greist et al,[41] 118 patients who had responded to 12 weeks' treatment with either sertraline or placebo

Table 9.5 Placebo-controlled continuation studies in OCD.

Author	Active treatment	No.	Duration (weeks)
Cottraux et al (1990)[39]	Fluvoxamine + exposure[a]	50	8
		44	24
		37	48
Katz et al (1990)[40]	Clomipramine[b]	110	[10+] 52
Tollefson et al (1994)[31]	Fluoxetine[b]	76	[13+] 24
Greist et al (1995)[41]	Sertraline[b]	118	[12+] 40

[a]Extended double-blind study.
[b]Double-blind continuation in selected acute-phase [x weeks] responders.

continued their ascribed treatment, double-blind, for 40 weeks. The patients maintained their improvements as long as they remained on active sertraline. Side effects improved over time, and compliance was good – only 13% of patients on sertraline dropped out of treatment prematurely during the extension phase. The 59 patients who completed this study were followed up for a second year on open-label sertraline, whereupon they showed additional clinical improvements.[37]

These results suggest treatment continues to be effective in the longer term.

How long should treatment continue?

Most patients are anxious to know how long they need to take their medication for. One way of tackling this question is to explore whether long-term continuation of pharmacotherapy provides ongoing protection against relapse. A particularly promising technique involves taking patients who have responded to the active drug and comparing their relapse rates following randomization to either continuous treatment or drug discontinuation.

The interpretation of discontinuation studies is not always straightforward. The lack of agreed criteria for defining a relapse of OCD makes comparisons between the studies difficult. In addition, the studies cannot control against 'withdrawal' effects resulting from the abrupt discontinuation of the medication. Withdrawal effects are related to the pharmacological properties of the treatment agent, and are believed to complicate clomipramine and paroxetine rather more than fluoxetine.[42] They can be difficult to distinguish from early signs of the re-emergence of OCD.

A series of controlled studies has shown that discontinuation of active treatment is associated with a significantly greater likelihood of symptomatic relapse (Table 9.6), irrespective of the duration of the treatment (up

Table 9.6 Relapse prevention in OCD: double-blind discontinuation studies.

Study	Drug	Duration of prior drug treatment	Number in study	Follow-up after discontinuation (weeks)	Outcome of discontinuation
Yaryura-Tobias et al (1976)[43]	Clomipramine	4 or 6 wk	13	1	Worsening of OCD
Flament et al (1985)[44]	Clomipramine	5 wk	19[a]	5	Worsening of OCD
Pato et al (1988)[45]	Clomipramine	5–27 mo	18	7	94.4% relapsed
Leonard et al (1988)[46]	Clomipramine	17 mo	21[b]	5	89% relapsed
Dunbar et al (1995)[47]	Paroxetine	9 mo	104[c]	36	58.8% relapsed
Romano et al (1998)[48]	Fluoxetine	20 wk	71[c]	52	32% relapsed
Robinson et al (1999)[49]	Sertraline	52 wk	121[c]	28	35.4% relapsed

[a]In children.
[b]In children and adolescents.
[c]Survival analysis performed.

to 2 years).[45] For most compounds, symptoms emerged within only a few weeks of stopping medication. The earlier clomipramine discontinuation studies showed higher relapse rates, possibly related to stronger withdrawal effects. In the fluoxetine study the relapse rates were lower overall, and benefits of ongoing treatment were seen only in the group receiving the 60 mg fixed dose. The study by Dunbar et al showed a convincing advantage for a further 6 months of paroxetine treatment in patients who had already responded well to 9 months of open-label treatment.[47] The study by Robinson et al, which has not yet been published in full, looked at patients who had responded to a year's treatment with sertraline. Twenty-eight weeks after randomization, 12% of patients continuing on sertraline had relapsed, compared with over 35% on placebo.[49] Quality-of-life scores continued to improve in the patients continuing their sertraline, and deteriorated in the group switched to placebo.

Altogether, the data suggest that medication confers protection against relapse for as long as it is continued. We may conclude that treatment should be continued for unlimited periods. Discontinuation, if necessary, should be gradual to minimize withdrawal effects, and patients should be warned to look out for signs of emerging illness, whereupon reinstatement of the drug may achieve the same level of improvement, although this cannot be guaranteed.[50]

What is the best dose for long-term treatment?

There is little evidence to support dose reduction in the longer term, apart from one small study in which lowering the dose of clomipramine and fluvoxamine did not appear to increase the rates of relapse.[51] In the study by Romano et al,[48] the 60 mg daily dose of fluoxetine appeared the most effective over a 24-week extension phase. On the limited data currently available, most experts recommend continuing treatment at the effective dose, and the adage 'the dose that gets you well, keeps you well' probably applies.

Other drugs in OCD

Although SRIs are impressively effective treatments for OCD, a substantial minority of cases, estimated at up to 30%, do not respond well. Attention has turned, therefore, to the investigation of alternative agents. So far, there is little evidence supporting the role of other forms of medication in OCD. A small preliminary analysis suggested that mianserin might be effective, but the definitive results were never published.[52] One small placebo-controlled study found promising results with clonazepam,[53] another with L-tryptophan.[54] The finding of no difference between phenelzine and clomipamine, in an underpowered study that lacked a placebo,[55] was contradicted by the negative placebo-controlled phenelzine-trial by Jenike et al.[2] Clorgyline has also been shown to be less effective than clomipramine,[56] implying that there is no role for monoamine oxidase inhibitors in OCD. The results for buspirone have been similarly unconvincing.

Conclusion

Treatment with serotonin reuptake inhibitors effects a slow, gradual improvement in OCD for the majority of patients. The selective SRIs are better tolerated than clomipramine. Treatment needs to be long term, and doses should be titrated upwards to achieve optimal results. The response to medication can be summarized as follows:

- Early onset of response may be hard to detect.
- Slow, gradual improvements take place over weeks and months.
- Comprehensive improvement in obsessions, compulsions and mood is observed.
- Effects are sustained as long as treatment is continued.
- Long-term treatment protects against relapse.
- Inadequate response occurs in a significant minority of cases.

References

1 Goodman W, Price L, Delgado P et al, Specificity of serotonin reuptake inhibitors in the treatment of obsessive compulsive disorder: comparison of fluoxamine and desipramine, *Arch Gen Psychiatry* (1990) **47**:577–85.

2 Jenike MA, Baer L, Minichiello WE et al, Placebo-controlled trial of fluoxetine and phenelzine for obsessive-compulsive disorder, *American Journal of Psychiatry*, (1997) **154**:1261–4.

3 Zohar J, Chopra M, Sasson Y et al, Psychopharmacology of obsessive compulsive disorder? *World J Biol Psychiatry* (2000) **1**(2):92–100.

4 McDougle CJ, Goodman WK, Leckman J et al, Haloperidol addition in fluvoxamine-refractory

obsessive compulsive disorder, *Arch Gen Psychiatry* (1994) **51**: 302–8.

5 McDougle CJ, Epperson CN, Pelton GH et al, A double-blind, placebo-controlled study of risperidone addition in serotonin reuptake inhibitor-refractory obsessive compulsive disorder, *Arch Gen Psychiatry* (2000) **57**(8):794–801.

6 Mundo E, Guglielmo E, Bellodi L, Effect of adjuvant pindolol on the antiobsessional response to fluvoxamine: a double-blind, placebo-controlled study, *Int Clin Psychopharmacol* (1998) **13**(5): 219–24.

7 Dannon PN, Sasson Y, Hirschmann S et al, Pindolol augmentation in treatment resistant

obsessive compulsive disorder: a double-blind placebo-controlled trial, *Eur Neuropsychopharmacol* (2000) **10**(3):165–9.

8 Fineberg NA, Roberts A, Montgomery SA et al, Brain 5-HT function in obsessive-compulsive disorder. Prolactin responses to D-fenfluramine, *Br J Psychiatry* (1997) **171:**280–2.

9 Fernandez CE, Lopez-Ibor JJ, Monochlorimipramine in the treatment of psychiatric patients resistant to other therapies, *Actas Luso Esp Neurol Psiquiatr Cienc Afines* (1967) **26**:119–47.

10 Reynghe De Voxrie GV, Anafranil (G34586) in obsessive neurosis, *Acta Neurol Belg* (1968) **68**:787–92.

11 Montgomery SA, Clomipramine in obsessional neurosis; a placebo-controlled trial, *Pharmacol Med* (1980) **1**:189–92.

12 De Veaugh-Geiss J, Landau P, Katz R, Treatment of obsessive compulsive disorder with clomipramine, *Psychiatry Annals* (1989) **19**:97–101.

13 Goodman WK, Price LH, Rasmussen SA et al, The Yale-Brown Obsessive-Compulsive Scale I: development, use, and reliability, *Arch Gen Psychiatry* (1984) **46**:1006–11.

14 Piccinelli M, Pini S, Bellantuono C et al, Efficacy of drug treatment in obsessive compulsive disorder, *Br J Psychiatry* (1995) **166**:424–43.

15 Piggott TA, Pato MT, Bernstein SE et al, Controlled comparison of clomipramine and fluoxetine in the treatment of obsessive compulsive disorder, *Arch Gen Psychiatry* (1990) **144**:1543–8.

16 Lopez-Ibor JJ, Saiz J, Cottraux J et al, Double-blind comparison of fluoxetine versus clomipramine in the treatment of obsessive compulsive disorder, *Eur Neuropsy-chopharmacol* (1996) **6**(2):111–18.

17 Smeraldi E, Ergovesi S, Bianchi I et al, Fluvoxamine versus clomipramine treatment in obsessive compulsive disorder: a preliminary study, *New Trends Exper Clin Psychiatry* (1992) **8**(2):63–5.

18 Freeman CPL, Trimble MR, Deakin JFW et al, Fluvoxamine versus clomipramine in the treatment of obsessive compulsive disorder. A multicentre, randomised, double-blind parallel group comparison, *J Clin Psychiatry* (1994) **55**(7):301–5.

19 Koran LM, McElroy SL, Davidson JRT et al, Fluvoxamine versus clomipramine for obsessive compulsive disorder: a double-blind comparison, *J Clin Psychopharmacol* (1996) **16**(2):121–9.

20 Milanfranchi A, Ravagli S, Lensi P et al, A double-blind study of fluvoxamine and clomipramine in the treatment of obsessive-compulsive disorder. *Int Clin Psychopharmacol* (1997) **12**:131–6.

21 Rouillon F, A double-blind comparison of fluvoxamine and clomipramine in OCD, *Eur Neuropsychopharmacol* (1998) **8**(2):S260–1.

22 Zohar J, Judge R, Paroxetine versus clomipramine in the treatment of obsessive compulsive disorder. *Br J Psychiatry* (1996) **169**:468–74.

23 Bisserbe JC, Lane RM, Flament MF et al, A double-blind comparison of sertraline and clomipramine in outpatients with obsessive compulsive disorder, *Eur Psychiatry* (1997) **153**:1450–4.

24 Pidrman V, Tuma I, Citalopram versus clomipramine in double-blind therapy of obsessive compulsive disorder, *Abstracts 11th Congress European College of Neuropsychopharmacology*, Oct 31–Nov 4, Paris, 1998.

25 Montgomery SA, Fineberg N, Montgomery DB, The efficacy of serotonergic drugs in OCD-power calculations compared with placebo. In: Montgomery SA, Goodman WK, Goeting N, eds, *Current Approaches: Obsessive Compulsive Disorder* (Ashford Duphar: Southampton, 1990) 54–63.

26 Hoehn-Saric R, Harrison W, Clary C, Obsessive compulsive disorder with comorbid major depression: a comparison of sertraline and desipramine treatment. Poster presented at 10th ECNP, Vienna, Austria.

27 Kejsers G, Hooddiun C, Schaap CP, Predictors of treatment outcome in the behavioural treatment of obsessive compulsive disorder, *Br J Psychiatry* (1994) **165**: 781–6.

28 Hohagen F, Winkelmann G, Rasche-Rauchle H et al, Combination of behaviour therapy with fluvoxamine in comparison with behaviour therapy and placebo. Results of a multicentre study, *Br J Psychiatry* (1998) **173**:71–8.

29 Fineberg NA, Roberts A, Montgomery SA, Are higher doses more effective in OCD? *Eur Neuropsychopharmacol* (1994) **4**(3): 264–5.

30 Montgomery SA, McIntyre A, Osterheider M et al, A double-blind placebo-controlled study of fluoxetine inpatients with DSM-III-R obsessive compulsive disorder. The Lilly European OCD Study Group, Eur Neuropsychopharmacol (1993) **3**:143–52.

31 Tollerfson G, Rampey A, Potvin J et al, A multicentive investigation of fixed-dose fluoxetine in the treatment of obsessive compulsive disorder, *Archives of General Psychiatry* (1994) **51**:559–67.

32 Greist J, Chouinard G, Duboff E et al, Double-blind parallel comparison of three dosages of sertraline and placebo in outpatients with obsessive compulsive disorder, *Arch Gen Psychiatry* (1995) **52**:289–95.

33 Wheadon D, Bushnell W, Steiner M, A fixed dose comparison of 20, 40 or 60 mg paroxetine to placebo in the treatment of obsessive compulsive disorder. Poster presented at the Annual Meeting of the American College of Neuropsychopharmacology, Honolulu, Hawaii (1993).

34 Montgomery SA, Citalopram treatment of obsessive compulsive disorder: results from a double-blind, placebo-controlled trial. Poster presented at the 37th Annual Meeting of the American College of Neuropsychopharmacology, Las Croaloas, Puerto Rico, December 1998.

35 Wood A, Tollefson GD, Burkitt M. Pharmacotherapy of obsessive compulsive disorder – experience with fluoxetine, *Int Clin Psychopharmacol* (1993) **8**:301–6.

36 Stahl S, *Psychopharmacology of Antidepressants* (Martin Dunitz: London, 1997) 56–8.

37 Rasmussen S, Hackett E, DuBoff E et al, A 2-year study of sertraline in the treatment of obsessive-compulsive disorder, *Int Clin Psychopharmacol* (1997) **12**: 309–16.

38 Wagner KD, March J, Landau P et al, Safety and efficacy of sertraline in long-term paediatric OCD treatment: a multicentre study. Presented at the 39th Annual Meeting of the New Clinical Drug Evaluation Unit, Boca Raton, Fla, 1999.

39 Cottraux J, Mollard E, Bouvard M et al, A controlled study of fluvoxamine and exposure in obsessive compulsive disorders, *Int Clin Psychopharmacol* (1990) **5**: 17–30.

40 Katz RJ, De Veaugh-Geiss J, Landau P, Clomipramine in obsessive-compulsive disorder, *Biol Psychiatry* (1990) **18**:401–4.

41 Greist J, Jefferson J, Kobak K et al, A one year double blind placebo-controlled fixed dose study of sertraline in the treatment of obsessive compulsive disorder, *International Clinical Psychopharmacology* (1995) **10**: 57–65.

42 Sechter D, Lane R, Continuation therapy with selective serotonin reuptake inhibitors, *J Ser Res* (1997) **4**:65–113.

43 Yaryura-Tobias JA, Neziroglu F, Bergman L, Clomipramine for obsessive-compulsive neurosis: an organic approach, *Curr Therapeutics Res* (1976) **20**:541–8.

44 Flament MF, Rapoport JL, Berg CJ, Clomipramine treatment of childhood OCD: a double-blind controlled study, *Arch Gen Psychiatry* (1985) **42**:977–83.

45 Pato MT, Zohar-Kadouch R, Zohar J, Return of symptoms after discontinuation of clomipramine in patients with obsessive compulsive disorder, *Am J Psychiatry* (1988) **145**:211–14.

46 Leonard H, Swedo S, Rapoport J et al, Treatment of childhood obsessive compulsive disorder with clomipramine and desmethylimipramine: a double blind crossover comparison, *Psychopharmacol Bull* (1988) **24**(1): 93–5.

47 Dunbar G, Steiner M, Bushnell WD et al, Long-term treatment and prevention of relapse of obsessive compulsive disorder with paroxetine, *Eur Neuropsychopharmacol* (1995) **5**:372.

48 Romano S, Goodman WK, Tamura T et al, Long-term treatment of obsessive-compulsive disorder following acute response: a comparison of fluoxetine versus placebo, *Eur Neuropsychopharmacol* (1998) **8**(suppl. 2):261.

49 Robinson D, Kiev A, Hackett E et al, Sertraline in long-term OCD treatment: results of a multicentre study. Presented at the XI World Congress of Psychiatry, Hamburg, 1999.

50 Ravizza L, Maina G, Bogetto F et al, Long-term treatment of obsessive compulsive disorder, *CNS Drugs* (1998) **10**(4):247–55.

51 Mundo E, Bareggi SR, Pirola R et al, Long-term pharmacotherapy of obsessive compulsive disorder: a double-blind controlled study, *J Clin Psychopharmacol* (1997) **17**:4–10.

52 Jaskari MO, Observations on mianserin in the treatment of obsessive neuroses, *Curr Med Res Opin* **6**:128–31.

53 Hewlett WA, Vinogradov S, Agras WS, Clomipramine, clonazepam and clonidine treatment of obsessive-compulsive disorder, *J Clin Psychopharmacol* (1992) **12**:420–30.

54 Montgomery SA, Fineberg NA, Montgomery DB et al, L-tryptophan in obsessive compulsive disorder – a placebo-controlled study, *Eur Neuropsychopharmacol* (1992) **2**(suppl. 2):384.

55 Vallejo J, Olivares J, Marcos TI et al, Clomipramine versus phenelzine in obsessive compulsive disorder. A controlled clinical trial, *Br J Psychiatry* (1992) **161**: 665–70.

56 Insel TR, Murphy DL, Cohen RM et al, Obsessive-compulsive disorder – a double-blind trial of clomipramine and clorgyline, *Arch Gen Psychiatry* (1983) **40**: 605–12.

10
Psychotherapy in OCD

Andreas Broocks and Fritz Hohagen

For decades, obsessive compulsive disorder (OCD) was considered to be a fascinating but treatment-refractory mental condition. Conventional pharmacological approaches as well as psychodynamic therapy failed to achieve satisfactory improvements in obsessive compulsive symptomatology.[1] The first major advances in the treatment of OCD came from two different approaches. Clomipramine, which differs from other tricyclic antidepressants by its potent inhibition of serotonin reuptake, proved to exert specific antiobsessional effects. At the same time, the introduction of special cognitive-behavioral techniques began to improve the prognosis of OCD continuously. In subsequent years, many studies have shown that behavior therapy, especially exposure with response prevention, and selective serotonin reuptake inhibitors (SSRIs) reduce obsessive compulsive symptoms significantly.[2–6] Nevertheless, several questions remain open for discussion and further research. This article reviews different psychotherapeutic approaches in the treatment of OCD such as exposure therapy, cognitive techniques, multimodal behavioral therapy, and group therapy. In addition, the question of combined behavioral and pharmacotherapeutic treatment is discussed, and suggestions for further research are given.

Early treatment approaches

The first psychological interventions in the treatment of OCD were exposure techniques such as systematic desensitization and reinforcement procedures including aversion. Unfortunately, these therapies were not very effective.[7,8] The first approach, which in fact resembled current forms of imaginative and in vivo exposure, was the so-called paradoxical intention: in vivo confrontation with symptom-inducing stimuli was coupled with instructions to elaborate the obsessional material. These early approaches helped to advance the development of the modern exposure and response prevention technique which has proved to be highly effective. Early cognitive interventions such as thought-stopping were only examined in case reports or in uncontrolled studies without any long-term documentation of therapy success.

Exposure and response prevention

Meyer's case report is, to our knowledge, the first description of a successful behavioral treatment characterized by prolonged exposure to obsessional cues and – at the same time – strict prevention of responses.[9] This finding was corroborated in two further open studies which additionally demonstrated a surprisingly low relapse rate at 5-year follow-up. Meanwhile, exposure/response prevention has been compared with various control treatments including relaxation, anxiety management training, and pill placebo,[10] leading to further evidence for the efficacy of this procedure. Current exposure/response prevention programs usually combine in vivo exercises of exposure to feared stimuli with imaginative exposure.[11] Repeated prolonged exposure leads to a psychophysiological habituation process, which also affects irrational beliefs held by the patient. Most therapists use gradual exposure which seems to be associated with better acceptance by the patients. Flooding has not been observed to be better than a gradual approach.[7] Because motivation is crucial for a successful therapy, we prefer a hierarchy-oriented increase of exposure intensity. We also recommend the addition of imaginal exposure to in vivo exposure/response prevention, which has shown to be advantageous in clinical studies.[11] In some patients, in vivo exposure exercises are not possible, because their obsessional fears consist of unrealistic disastrous events; therefore, imaginal exposure is a key element of treatment in these patients. It is crucial that the duration of the exposure exercise continues at least until the patient experiences a decrease of the induced distress. The time needed to achieve sufficient habituation varies from patient to patient and will often require 90 minutes or more.[12] Some researchers have reported excellent results with a high-frequency treatment involving daily sessions, but favorable outcomes have also been gained with a session frequency of once per week.[13,14] In an inpatient treatment program patients with severe symptoms and those who exhibited considerable resistance to exposure were observed to benefit from a more intensive regimen.

Although there is only sparse evidence from clinical studies that therapist-assisted exposure is more potent than self-exposure, clinical experience suggests that patients will expose themselves to feared situations more readily in the presence of a therapist. In addition, patients are asked to conduct self-directed exposure exercises between these guided sessions. Importantly, patients should not be stopped from performing their rituals by physical prevention as described in the early studies of Meyer and co-workers. Instead, the therapist will give instructions and encouragement to support the patient's own decision not to perform compulsive behaviors.[15] Therapists should also be alert in order to detect and restrain covert neutralizing thoughts.[16] Alternative activities have to be practised for situations characterized by strong urges to indulge in obsessive compulsive behavior. In general, it will be helpful to find a friend or a family member who is able to provide co-therapeutic functions; this person must be trained in ways of supporting the patient between sessions in order to achieve adequate exposure. High emotional arousal is usually experienced as anxiety. However, some patients will describe their emotions during exposure as anger, aggression or depression. Irrespective of these emotional variations, the patient has the task of describing precisely the experienced emotions and the accompanying cognitions. This description is the basis of the cognitive restructuring which most therapists view as an important component of successful exposure.

Most studies that have examined the efficacy of exposure therapy for OCD also included response prevention techniques, thus confounding the effects of the single procedures. To separate these effects, Foa et al randomly assigned patients with compulsive washing to treatment by exposure only, response prevention only, or their combination (exposure/response prevention).[17] Results showed that the combined treatment was superior to the single treatments on most symptom measures.[17]

In summary, despite promising results from new cognitive approaches, exposure/response prevention still has the key role in the treatment of OCD. Foa and Kozak reviewed 12 outcome studies using exposure/response prevention ($n = 330$), and found that an average of 83% of treatment completers were classified as responders immediately after treatment.[18] In 16 studies reporting long-term outcome ($n = 376$) 76% of the patients were responders; the mean follow-up interval in the latter group of studies was 29 months. Several meta-analytic studies have detected large effect sizes for exposure/response prevention with OCD in adults (>1.0).[18]

Cognitive approaches in the treatment of OCD

In recent years, cognitive approaches have been proposed for the treatment of OCD, especially obsessional ruminations.[19,20] Cognitive therapy is thought to work by altering both strongly held beliefs associated with OCD symptoms and interpretations of intrusive mental experiences. Following the work of Rachman and Hodgson,[21] Salkovskis and co-workers distinguished between anxiety-producing thoughts and secondary neutralizing thoughts.[16,22] They proposed exposure techniques by thought evocation or listening to a 'loop tape' of the anxiety-provoking thought in the patient's own voice followed by response prevention (i.e. no overt or covert neutralizing or avoidance behavior). Additionally, a cognitive model of OCD was developed based on the general model as applied to anxiety disorders. The cognitive-behavioral theory of OCD proposes that obsessional thoughts and normal intrusive thoughts do not in themselves differ.[23,24] The difference lies in how the obsessional patient interprets the occurrence and/or content of the intrusions. According to the cognitive hypothesis, obsessional problems occur when intrusive cognitions are interpreted as an indication that the person may be, may have been, or may come to be responsible for harm or its prevention.[20,25] According to Salkovskis, this specific interpretation of the occurrence and content of intrusive thoughts – responsibility for harm to oneself or other people – links intrusions with both the discomfort experienced and the neutralizing (compulsive) behaviors whether overt or covert. Neutralizing and avoidance behavior, a tendency to overfocus attention on the contents of one's own mind, and negative mood can all interact, in the context of the general cognitive theory, to maintain the negative belief concerning responsibility.[22] Cognitive therapy seeks to change responsibility beliefs and appraisals and thereby to reduce distress and eliminate neutralizing responses, which usually occur as covert neutralizing (mental) rituals. In contrast to the fears of patients suffering from panic disorder or social phobia, the catastrophes feared by OCD patients usually lie further in the future; therefore, disconfirmation is much less useful as a strategy. Much depends on a process in which the patient and the therapist develop a non-threatening explanation of the problem. This alternative account reminds the patient that there are at least two possible explanations for the problem: it is possible that there really is a danger of causing harm or not preventing negative incidents; on the other hand there might only be excessive worry about possible harm leading to constant anxiety and concern.

Many obsessional patients try to suppress their anxiety-laden thoughts. Some of these patients believe that they are not overwhelmed by their obsessional thoughts only because of their constant resistance or because of distraction techniques. In such a situation cognitive therapists would introduce behavioral experiments. In this example, the patient would be asked to keep a diary record of the frequency and intensity of the obsessional thought under two opposite conditions: on the first day every attempt should be made to distract attention from the thought, and on the other day all thoughts should be allowed to come and go without suppressing them. It is also important to help patients to identify and to modify underlying general assumptions which might represent the roots of the more overt dysfunctional thoughts. As in other anxiety disorders, the general style of therapy is that of guided discovery. Further details of the cognitive treatment of obsessions including the use of loop tapes are described by Salkovskis et al.[22]

A number of published case reports in case series provide evidence for the clinical effectiveness of the cognitive approach.[19,26] More recently, Freeston reported the results of a controlled trial in which cognitive-behavioral therapy (CBT) was significantly superior in comparison with a waiting-list control group.[27] Treatment effects persisted at 6-month follow-up, Schwartz has proposed a cognitive-biobehavioral self-treatment for OCD.[28] This integrates the results of neuroimaging research into the cognitive approach based on the literature on the behavioral neurobiology of the basal ganglia. It is founded on the assumption that OCD symptoms are related to a malfunction in cortical circuit activation in the fronto-striatal system; therefore, activation of an alternative circuit through the focused performance of a familiar alternative behavior might over time ameliorate the discomfort related to the faulty brain mechanism. In a four-step process, the OCD patient learns to identify his or her obsessions and compulsions, to label them as such ('It's not me, it is my OCD'), and to attribute them to abnormal activity of the frontostriatal system ('relabel, reattribute, refocus, revalue'). While 'working around OCD symptoms', patients learn new adaptive responses to intrusive OCD thoughts and urges. They are tutored to become increasingly aware of avoidant behaviors and to use treatment techniques to perform previously avoided behaviors. As a result of this systematic change in behavioral responses to OCD symptoms, patients come to revalue the intrusive thoughts and urges as much less important and noteworthy. Fear and anxiety associated with OCD symptoms gradually fade.[28]

Since these cognitive approaches have to varying extents included exposure techniques, the question remains whether pure cognitive therapy is equivalent to exposure therapy in the treatment of OCD, or whether the addition of cognitive techniques can improve the results of exposure therapy. The efficacy of rational emotive therapy (RET), a cognitive therapy program that focuses on irrational beliefs, has been examined by Emmelkamp et al.[29] Patients were randomly assigned to RET or to exposure/response prevention, the RET focused on irrational thoughts that caused negative feelings and the modification of these thoughts by cognitive techniques in order to reduce anxiety and the urge to perform rituals. At the end of the treatment, both groups showed comparable improvements. Van Oppen et al compared the efficacy of self-controlled exposure/response prevention and a cognitive intervention developed to correct specific cognitive distortions. At the end of the treatment period, OCD symptom reductions of 20% were observed for cognitive therapy and 23% for exposure/response prevention.[30] This study, however, compared cognitive techniques with self-help exposure, the least effective version of exposure; therapist-guided exposure, which may be more efficacious, was not included. James and Blackburn presented a meta-analysis of 15 published studies of cognitive therapy in OCD. They did not find a significant additional effect ascribable to cognitive therapy.[31]

Most studies comparing exposure/response prevention to variants of cognitive therapy are limited by the fact that the behavioral exercises are not applied in the intensity and/or frequency necessary to achieve optimal effects. Cottraux and co-workers compared cognitive therapy with intensive behavioral therapy in 64 outpatients in a multicenter study.[32] Group 1 received twenty 1-hour sessions of cognitive therapy over 16 weeks. Group 2 received a 4-week intensive treatment with two sessions of 2 hours' duration per week and a 12-week maintenance phase with booster sessions. The behavioral therapy program included imaginal and in vivo exposure with response prevention during the sessions, and homework. Preliminary data indicate that there were no significant differences between the two treatment groups. This study suggests that cognitive therapy is as effective as exposure therapy. However, recent meta-analytic findings suggest that cognitive therapies which also use 'behavioral experiments' are superior to pure cognitive approaches.[33] On the other hand, 'pure' exposure/response prevention is a theoretical construct, because dysfunctional thinking and irrational beliefs are usually discussed during exposure sessions. It is likely that one of the central mechanisms explaining the efficacy of exposure is the correction of false beliefs. Accordingly, cognitive therapy will always include behavioral experiments as an important tool for cognitive restructuring.[7] Therefore, in clinical practice, it seems justified to use the term 'cognitive-behavioral therapy' (CBT) for all of these approaches.

Multimodal cognitive-behavioral therapy

Unfortunately, at least 25% of OCD patients do not comply with cognitive behavioral therapy.[34] In addition to those who drop out, 20–30% do not respond sufficiently. Thus, a considerable number of patients are in need of further support.[35] Interestingly, biographies of OCD patients show that at least half of them suffer from anxiety problems, low self-esteem, social deficits, and more or less latent aggression resulting in marked problems in daily life conduct.[36] To treat these patients more effectively, there is an increasing interest in multimodal CBT programs. This treatment approach analyzes and treats early social deficits, reduced tolerance for intensive emotions, and reduced emotional awareness. It deals with deficits in problem-solving and self-initiated alternative behaviors as well as interpersonal problems. Principally, it also uses symptom-directed interventions, i.e. cognitive techniques and exposure with response prevention. Prior to developing the first treatment plan in collaboration with the patient, it is helpful to check whether the following assessments have already been made from the information gained in the first few sessions with the patient: internal or external motivation for treatment and change, other interpersonal or financial problems, biographical analysis in order to identify factors that have triggered or maintained the OCD symptomatology, and functional analysis of compulsive or obsessional symptoms. It is also important to discuss the consequences for daily life when most of the OCD symptoms have disappeared. This rather complex analysis may lead to quite different treatment plans: in 'uncomplicated' cases, symptom-directed treatment might be the only therapeutic intervention; other patients will additionally require techniques in order to reduce triggering and maintaining factors. More severely affected patients might need the full armoury of the multimodal approach: symptom-directed cognitive and exposure techniques, deficit-directed procedures such as social skills training, problem-solving skills, self-induced alternative behaviors, and interventions aiming to increase motivation for change. This approach also tries to reduce perfectionism, striving for absolute security and predictability of future events. In severe cases, complex combinations of multimodal interventions are often needed, including marital or family interventions as well as individual or group treatments. In addition to symptom reduction, in multimodal CBT patients are trained to improve their awareness of unresolved problems, their behavioural deficits, and their personal resources and abilities that can be activated for significant progress in daily life conduct.

Multimodal CBT has been shown to be effective, with very low drop-out rates in severely ill inpatients and outpatients.[37,38] Furthermore, its long-term efficacy has been demonstrated in follow-up studies in unselected patients.[38] Whether multimodal behavioral therapy is superior to exposure therapy alone, and whether it is appropriate to treat refusers, drop-outs, and non-responders to conventional exposure therapy with response prevention, are still open questions. Furthermore, the impact of different health-care systems on patient selection has to be taken into consideration. While most of the studies carried out in the USA involved motivated outpatients, European studies have been carried out with patients referred to psychiatry departments;[37–39] these patients often have low motivation to change behavior. A health-care system that covers all treatment costs including repeated hospital treatments of variable length might also impair the motivation to change obsessive compulsive behavior in some patients. Thus, increasing motivation for behavioral change is an important part of multimodal behavioral therapy; it may make this approach useful for OCD patients who drop out or refuse to undergo exposure therapy alone.

Group therapy

The different variations of CBT discussed so far have well-established efficacy for the treatment of OCD. However, the lack of experienced therapists and the cost of multiple individual treatment sessions often preclude its use and raise the question of whether these interventions could be applied successfully in the form of group therapy. Evidence for the clinical efficacy of group therapy derives from several studies.[40–42] It was reported that group therapy reduced distress caused by OCD symptoms, general depression, and anxiety by the end of treatment, although patients receiving individual behavioral therapy demonstrated faster reductions in OCD symptom severity.[41,42] A 6-month follow-up showed that treated participants were able to maintain their gains. Another recent study added more evidence for the clinical efficacy of group therapy treatment.[43] However, patients in both studies were moderately ill and the decrease in Yale–Brown Obsessive Compulsive Scale (Y–BOCS, see Appendix 1, p. 183) values was somewhat lower after 12 weeks of treatment compared with individual treatment in more severely ill OCD patients.[44,45] Thus, further research is needed to investigate whether group therapy is as effective as individual therapy in the treatment of OCD patients.

Combination of CBT and medication

Only a few studies have investigated whether the combination of pharmacotherapy with CBT is superior to CBT alone. Furthermore, few data are available on the differential indication for pharmacotherapy, CBT, or combined treatment. Marks et al have compared the combination of clomipramine plus exposure in vivo with clomipramine and exposure separately.[46] When added to exposure therapy, clomipramine treatment improved some measures of rituals and depression significantly more than placebo medication during 7 weeks of self-exposure instructions. This effect was transient and disappeared as drug treatment and exposure were continued for a further 15 weeks. The authors concluded that clomipramine had a limited adjuvant role.[46] The results from another study indicated that although imipramine improved depressive symptoms in depressed patients with OCD, it did not affect obsessive compulsive symptoms and did not potentiate the antiobsessional effects of behavior therapy.[44] Cottraux et al compared exposure therapy, fluvoxamine, and combination treatment in patients with OCD.[32] They reported a drug effect on rituals at week 8 and on depression at week 24. Both effects disappeared at week 48 and at the 18-month follow-up; patients as a whole remained improved with no between-group differences. The sequential combination of fluvoxamine with cognitive therapy or exposure in vivo with response prevention was not superior to either cognitive therapy or exposure alone.[45] Khanna and co-workers conducted a study to evaluate the differences between treatment with fluoxetine alone versus fluoxetine plus exposure and response prevention in 40 previously untreated patients with OCD.[47] They concluded that exposure and response prevention may have a limited role in the initial treatment of

OCD. Hohagen et al investigated whether the combination of multimodal CBT with fluvoxamine is superior to CBT and placebo in the acute treatment of severely ill inpatients with OCD.[37] This study also looked at whether the pharmacologic treatment of secondary depression improves the treatment outcome of obsessive and compulsive symptoms. Both groups showed a highly significant symptom reduction after treatment. There were no significant differences between the groups concerning compulsions. Obsessions were significantly more reduced in the fluvoxamine–CBT group than in the placebo–CBT group. Furthermore, the fluvoxamine–CBT group showed a significantly higher response rate (87.5% versus 60%) according to the previously defined response criterion (>35% symptom reduction in the Y–BOCS scores, see Appendix 1, p. 183). Severely depressed patients with OCD receiving CBT plus fluvoxamine had a significantly better treatment outcome (Y–BOCS scores, see Appendix 1, p. 183) than severely depressed OCD patients receiving CBT plus placebo. The authors concluded that differential analysis of the clinical syndrome of OCD suggests different treatment strategies. When compulsions dominate the clinical picture, CBT alone seems to be sufficient to treat patients effectively. If the patients suffer predominantly from obsessions, then addition of SSRI therapy to CBT may improve treatment outcome. If the patients suffer from secondary depression, SSRIs seem to enhance the treatment outcome of OCD significantly and should be added to CBT. Furthermore, from the literature it can be concluded that SSRIs should be combined with a neuroleptic, if a tic disorder is present in addition to OCD.[48] Unfortunately, there is a high relapse rate of around 70–80% after discontinuation of medication.[49,50] A clinical study is in progress to find out to what extent this relapse rate can be reduced by concomitant CBT.

Predictors of treatment outcome

The identification of prognostic variables associated with treatment failure or success could lead to modified treatment programs. Most data on predictors of treatment outcome are derived from psychopharmacologic studies.[51] Studies investigating prognostic factors for CBT have identified the following negative predictors: high OCD severity at the beginning of treatment;[35,52] severe depression;[8,35,37,53] overvalued or fixed obsessive ideation;[54] unemployment; [55,56] comorbidity with personality disorder;[57–59] and lack of motivation for treatment.[52] The presence of hoarding obsessions and compulsions was also associated with poorer response to serotonin reuptake inhibitors.[60] Certain personality disorders, especially schizotypal and borderline conditions, have also been found related to poor response to serotonin reuptake inhibitors.[29,57] A 2-year follow-up study after multimodal inpatient treatment showed that treatment compliance was a predictor for long-term outcome. Patients who discontinued exposure therapy were more likely to be classified as non-responders (response defined as 35% symptom reduction in the Y–BOCS (see Appendix 1); F Hohagen et al, unpublished data). The importance of exposure therapy was also underlined by a study by De Araujo and co-workers.[15] The best predictor of good outcome at the end of treatment (week 9) and of follow-up (week 32) was early compliance in doing exposure homework within a week of starting treatment. These studies have been done in adult OCD patients. Predictors of CBT outcome have not been reported for child-hood OCD.

Future questions

Although the percentage of patients who refuse to participate in behavioral therapy is smaller in the multimodal approach when compared with the intensive exposure/response prevention treatment programs, the motivational background for this kind of avoidance behavior should be examined in greater depth in order to find new ways of overcoming these barriers to effective treatment. We also need studies in community-based treatment facilities to find out whether the excellent results from specialized centers can be obtained in other settings. The efficacy, acceptance and cost-effectiveness of short-term interventions for patients suffering from less severe forms of OCD need further improvement. Self-directed exposure using self-help manuals seems to be effective in a subgroup of OCD patients. More research is required to identify patients who are able to overcome their problems by pure self-help or manual-guided exposure strategies. The German Society for the Treatment of Obsessive Compulsive Disorder supports the foundation of self-help groups all over the country; the scientific evaluation concerning the therapeutic and health-economic potential of these groups is still at a preliminary stage.[61]

Another intriguing research field is the question whether neurobiological abnormalities associated with OCD can be modulated by effective treatment strategies. With cognitive-behavioral treatment, significant decreases in caudate glucose metabolism were found in treatment responders compared with non-responders. Pretreatment metabolic correlations between orbital cortex and caudate and between orbital cortex and thalamus were found, which decreased significantly with successful CBT.[62,63] Furthermore, the percentage change in the Y–BOCS score (see Appendix 1) was positively correlated with the percentage change in metabolism in the left orbital cortex.[63] It would be of great interest if parameters which (in comparison to positron emission tomography findings) can be more easily measured in clinical settings turn out to be predictors of treatment success or predictors of relapse at the end of a successful treatment.

Conclusion

In summary, the results of existing studies suggest that cognitive-behavioral therapy which includes exposure/response prevention and possibly other elements from the multimodal approach represents a treatment of choice for the majority of patients suffering from OCD. When CBT is not available or is rejected by the patient, or is ineffective, serotonergic medications are a therapeutic alternative with well-documented efficacy. Also, when the OCD is complicated by severe depression or when patients suffer predominantly from obsessions, pharmacotherapy is likely to improve the outcome of CBT. It is considered to be one of the major disadvantages of drug therapy that symptom reappearance generally occurs after tapering off the medication. However, in the authors' experience the long-term effects of CBT, demonstrated in several follow-up studies, also depend on the continuous practice of the newly adopted cognitive and behavioral strategies. Recurrence of OCD symptoms is likely when patients do not adhere to the newly adopted cognitive-behavioral habits because of motivational problems, acute life stress or depression. Despite all progress in treatment, OCD still is a chronic disorder which principally needs long-term treatment. However, it is a major advance that new, sophisticated cognitive-behavioral treatment programs enable many OCD patients to become their own experts in overcoming OCD-related symptoms and associated psychosocial impairments.

References

1 Greist JH, Treatment of obsessive compulsive disorder: psychotherapies, drugs, and other somatic treatment, *J Clin Psychiatry* (1990) 44–50; discussion 55–8.

2 Marks I, Behaviour therapy for obsessive-compulsive disorder: a decade of progress, *Can J Psychiatry* (1997) **42**(10):1021–7.

3 Greist JH, Jefferson JW, Pharmacotherapy for obsessive-compulsive disorder, *Br J Psychiatry* (1998) (suppl. 35): 64–70.

4 Pigott TA, Seay SM, A review of the efficacy of selective serotonin reuptake inhibitors in obsessive-compulsive disorder, *J Clin Psychiatry* (1999) **60**(2):101–6.

5 Mundo E, Bianchi L, Bellodi L, Efficacy of fluvoxamine, paroxetine, and citalopram in the treatment of obsessive-compulsive disorder: a single-blind study, *J Clin Psychopharmacol* (1997) **17**(4):267–71.

6 Rosenberg DR, Stewart CM, Fitzgerald KD, Tawile V, Carroll E, Paroxetine open-label treatment of pediatric outpatients with obsessive-compulsive disorder, *J Am Acad Child Adolesc Psychiatry* (1999) **38**(9):1180–5.

7 Minichiello WE, Baer L, Jenike MA, Behavior therapy for the treatment of obsessive-compulsive disorder: theory and practice, *Compr Psychiatry* (1988) **29**(2):123–37.

8   Foa EB, Failure in treating obsessive-compulsives, *Behav Res Ther* (1979) **17**(3):169–76.

9   Meyer V, Modifications of expectations in cases of obsessional rituals, *Behav Res Ther* (1966) **4**:273–80.

10 Kozak MJ, Liebowitz MR, Foa EB, Cognitive behavior therapy and pharmacotherapy for OCD. In: Goodman WK, ed., *Obsessive-Compulsive Disorder: Contemporary Issues in Treatment* (Harper: Washington, 1999).

11 Foa EB, Steketee G, Turner RM, Fischer SC, Effects of imaginal exposure to feared disasters in obsessive-compulsive checkers, *Behav Res Ther* (1980) **18**(5):449–55.

12 Foa EB, Chambless DL, Habituation of subjective anxiety during flooding in imagery, *Behav Res Ther* (1978) **16**(6):391–9.

13 Leonard HL, New developments in the treatment of obsessive-compulsive disorder, *J Clin Psychiatry* (1997) **14**(39):39–45; discussion 46–7.

14 Rapoport JL, Recent advances in obsessive-compulsive disorder [see comments], *Neuropsychopharmacology* (1991) **5**(1): 1–10.

15 De Araujo LA, Ito LM, Marks IM, Early compliance and other factors predicting outcome of exposure for obsessive-compulsive disorder, *Br J Psychiatry* (1996) **169**(6):747–52.

16 Salkovskis PM, Westbrook D, Davis J, Jeavons A, Gledhill A, Effects of neutralizing on intrusive thoughts: an experiment investigating the etiology of obsessive-compulsive disorder, *Behav Res Ther* (1997) **35**(3):211–19.

17 Foa EB, Steketee G, Milby JB, Differential effects of exposure and response prevention in obsessive-compulsive washers, *J Consult Clin Psychol* (1980) **48**(1):71–9.

18 Foa EB, Kozak MJ, Psychological treatment for OCD. In: Mavissakalian MR, Prien RF, eds, *Long-term Treatments of Anxiety Disorders* (American Psychiatric Press: Washington, 1996) 235–309.

19 Salkovskis PM, Understanding and treating obsessive-compulsive disorder, *Behav Res Ther* (1999) S29–52.

20 Salkovskis P, Shafran R, Rachman S, Freeston MH, Multiple pathways to inflated responsibility beliefs in obsessional problems: possible origins and implications for therapy and research, *Behav Res Ther* (1999) **37**(11):1055–72.

21 Rachman SJ, Hodgson RJ, *Obsessions and Compulsions* (Prentice-Hall: Englewood Cliffs, 1980).

22 Salkovskis PM, Forrester E, Richards C, Cognitive-behavioural approach to understanding obsessional thinking, *Br J Psychiatry* (1998) (suppl. 35):53–63.

23 Langlois F, Freeston MH, Ladouceur R, Differences and similarities between obsessive intrusive thoughts and worry in a non-clinical population: study 2, *Behav Res Ther* (2000) **38**(2): 175–89.

24 Langlois F, Freeston MH, Ladouceur R, Differences and similarities between obsessive intrusive thoughts and worry in a non-clinical population: study 1, *Behav Res Ther* (2000) **38**(2): 157–73.

25 Rheaume J, Freeston MH, Dugas MJ, Letarte H, Ladouceur R, Perfectionism, responsibility and obsessive-compulsive symptoms, *Behav Res Ther* (1995) **33**(7): 785–94.

26 Roth AD, Church JA, The use of revised habituation in the treatment of obsessive-compulsive

disorders, *Br J Clin Psychol* (1994) **3**:201–4.

27 Freeston MH, Ladouceur R, Gagnon F, Cognitive-behavioural treatment of obsessive thoughts: a controlled study, *J Consult Clin Psychol* (1997) **65**(3):405–13.

28 Schwartz JM, *Brain Lock* (Harper Collins: New York, 1996).

29 Emmelkamp PM, Beens H, Cognitive therapy with obsessive-compulsive disorder: a comparative evaluation, *Behav Res Ther* (1991) **29**(3):293–300.

30 Van Oppen P, de Haan E, van Balkom AJ, Spinhoven P, Hoogduin K, van Dyck R, Cognitive therapy and exposure in vivo in the treatment of obsessive compulsive disorder, *Behav Res Ther* (1995) **33**(4):379–90.

31 James IA, Blackburn IM, Cognitive therapy with obsessive-compulsive disorder [see comments], *Br J Psychiatry* (1995) **166**(4):444–50.

32 Cottraux J, Mollard E, Bouvard M, Marks I, Exposure therapy, fluvoxamine, or combination treatment in obsessive-compulsive disorder: one-year followup, *Psychiatry Res* (1993) **49**(1):63–75.

33 Abramowitz JS, Meta-analysis of psychological treatments in OCD, in press, 2001.

34 Schwartz JM, Neuroanatomical aspects of cognitive-behavioural therapy response in obsessive-compulsive disorder. An evolving perspective on brain and behaviour, *Br J Psychiatry* (1998) (suppl. 35):38–44.

35 Keijsers GP, Hoogduin CA, Schaap CP, Predictors of treatment outcome in the behavioural treatment of obsessive-compulsive disorder [see comments], *Br J Psychiatry* (1994) **165**(6):781–6.

36 Ehntholt KA, Salkovskis PM, Rimes KA, Obsessive-compulsive disorder, anxiety disorders, and self-esteem: an exploratory study, *Behav Res Ther* (1999) **37**(8):771–81.

37 Hohagen F, Winkelmann G, Rasche RH, Combination of behaviour therapy with fluvoxamine in comparison with behaviour therapy and placebo. Results of a multicentre study, *Br J Psychiatry* (1998) (suppl. 35):71–8.

38 Hand I, Out-patient, multi-modal behaviour therapy for obsessive-compulsive disorder, *Br J Psychiatry* (1998) (suppl. 35):45–52.

39 Munford PR, Hand I, Liberman RP, Psychosocial treatment for obsessive-compulsive disorder, *Psychiatry* (1994) **57**(2):142–52.

40 Krone KP, Himle JA, Nesse RM, A standardized behavioral group treatment program for obsessive-compulsive disorder: preliminary outcomes, *Behav Res Ther* (1991) **29**(6):627–31.

41 Fals-Stewart W, Lucente S, Behavioral group therapy with obsessive-compulsives: an overview, *Int J Group Psychother* (1994) **44**(1):35–51.

42 Fals-Stewart W, Marks AP, Schafer J, A comparison of behavioral group therapy and individual behavior therapy in treating obsessive-compulsive disorder [see comments], *J Nerv Ment Dis* (1993) **181**(3):189–93.

43 Van Noppen BI, Pato MT, Marsland R, Rasmussen SA, A time-limited behavioral group for treatment of obsessive-compulsive disorder, *J Psychother Pract Res* (1998) **7**(4):272–80.

44 Foa EB, Kozak MJ, Steketee GS, McCarthy PR, Treatment of depressive and obsessive-compulsive symptoms in OCD by imipramine and behaviour therapy, *Br J Clin Psychol* (1992) **4**:279–92.

45 Van Balkom AJ, de Haan E, van Oppen P, Spinhoven P, Hoogduin

KA, van Dyck R, Cognitive and behavioral therapies alone versus in combination with fluvoxamine in the treatment of obsessive compulsive disorder, *J Nerv Ment Dis* (1998) **186**(8):492–9.

46 Marks IM, Lelliott P, Basoglu M, Clomipramine, self-exposure and therapist-aided exposure for obsessive-compulsive rituals, *Br J Psychiatry* (1988) **152**:522–34.

47 Khanna S, Kumar R, The efficacy of addition of cognitive therapy to fluoxetine in the treatment of OCD. Third International OCD Conference, Madeira, Portugal, 1998.

48 McDougle CJ, Goodman WK, Leckman JF, Lee NC, Heninger GR, Price LH, Haloperidol addition in fluvoxamine-refractory obsessive-compulsive disorder. A double-blind, placebo-controlled study in patients with and without tics, *Arch Gen Psychiatry* (1994) **51**(4):302–8.

49 Pato MT, Hill JL, Murphy DL, A clomipramine dosage reduction study in the course of long-term treatment of obsessive-compulsive disorder patients, *Psychopharmacol Bull* (1990) **26**(2):211–14.

50 Pato MT, Zohar KR, Zohar J, Murphy DL, Return of symptoms after discontinuation of clomipramine in patients with obsessive-compulsive disorder, *Am J Psychiatry* (1988) **145**(12):1521–5.

51 DeVeaugh GJ, Katz R, Landau P, Goodman W, Rasmussen S, Clinical predictors of treatment response in obsessive compulsive disorder: exploratory analyses from multicenter trials of clomipramine, *Psychopharmacol Bull* (1990) **26**(1):54–9.

52 De Haan E, van Oppen P, van Balkom AJ, Spinhoven P, Hoogduin KA, van Dyck R, Prediction of outcome and early vs. late improvement in OCD patients treated with cognitive behaviour therapy and pharmacotherapy, *Acta Psychiatr Scand* (1997) **96**(5):354–61.

53 Foa EB, Grayson JB, Steketee GS, Doppelt HG, Turner RM, Latimer PR, Success and failure in the behavioral treatment of obsessive-compulsives, *J Consult Clin Psychol* (1983) **51**(2):287–97.

54 Kozak MJ, Foa EB, Obsessions, overvalued ideas, and delusions in obsessive-compulsive disorder, *Behav Res Ther* (1994) **32**(3):343–53.

55 Buchanan AW, Meng KS, Marks IM, What predicts improvement and compliance during the behavioral treatment of obsessive compulsive disorder? *Anxiety* (1996) **2**(1):22–7.

56 Castle DJ, Predictors of outcome in the behavioural treatment of OCD [letter; comment], *Br J Psychiatry* (1995) **166**(4):540–1.

57 Baer L, Jenike MA, Personality disorders in obsessive compulsive disorder, *Psychiatr Clin North Am* (1992) **15**(4):803–12.

58 Jenike MA, Baer L, Minichiello WE, Schwartz CE, Carey RJ, Concomitant obsessive-compulsive disorder and schizotypal personality disorder, *Am J Psychiatry* (1986) **143**(4):530–2.

59 Baer L, Jenike MA, Ricciardi JD, Standardized assessment of personality disorders in obsessive-compulsive disorder, *Arch Gen Psychiatry* (1990) **47**(9):826–30.

60 Mataix CD, Rauch SL, Manzo PA, Jenike MA, Baer L, Use of factor-analyzed symptom dimensions to predict outcome with serotonin reuptake inhibitors and placebo in the treatment of obsessive-compulsive disorder, *Am J Psychiatry* (1999) **156**(9):1409–16.

61 Münchau N, Hand I, Schaible R, Aufbau von Selbsthilfegruppen für Zwangskranke, *Verhaltenstherapie* (1996) **6**:143–61.

62 Baxter LJ, Schwartz JM, Bergman KS, Caudate glucose metabolic rate changes with both drug and behavior therapy for obsessive-compulsive disorder, *Arch Gen Psychiatry* (1992) **49**(9):681–9.

63 Schwartz JM, Stoessel PW, Baxter LJ, Martin KM, Phelps ME, Systematic changes in cerebral glucose metabolic rate after successful behavior modification treatment of obsessive-compulsive disorder, *Arch Gen Psychiatry* (1996) **53**(2):109–13.

11
Treatment of refractory OCD

Christopher J McDougle and Kelda H Walsh

The effectiveness of potent serotonin reuptake inhibitors (SRIs) and exposure with response prevention behavior therapy is now well established in the treatment of obsessive compulsive disorder (OCD). Despite these advances, nearly 40–60% of patients experience minimal to no improvement in symptoms with these treatments. Furthermore, in patients who do respond to SRI or behavior modification treatment, the degree of improvement is typically incomplete; few patients experience full symptom remission.[1]

Most large-scale, controlled studies of SRIs in OCD have defined treatment response by a 25–35% decrease from baseline on the total score of the Yale–Brown Obsessive Compulsive Scale (Y-BOCS, see Appendix 1, p. 183).[2,3] This magnitude of change typically results in significant improvement in function; however, interfering symptoms usually persist. Others have required that this criterion be met, along with a categorical response of 'much improved' or 'very much improved' on the global improvement item of the Clinical Global Impression (CGI) scale. In some studies, 'marked responders' have been patients who have met both of these response criteria, whereas 'partial responders' have been patients who have met one or the other criterion. Patients who demonstrate only a partial response or are unimproved following 10–12 week trials of two different selective SRIs (SSRIs) and the non-selective SRI clomipramine at adequate dosages, and who have shown no improvement with at least 20–30 hours of documented exposure with response prevention, should be considered for the alternative treatment approaches described in this chapter.

Results from controlled and uncontrolled investigations of various somatic interventions for patients with 'treatment-refractory' OCD have been published. These treatments have included the use of standard pharmacologic agents in higher dosages or administered via an alternative route (e.g. intravenous rather than oral clomipramine), combination drug treatment strategies, and the use of novel compounds. Studies of electroconvulsive therapy, repetitive transcranial magnetic stimulation and neurosurgery have also been conducted. This chapter will briefly review these data.

High-dose SRIs

Controlled studies of SSRIs administered in doses greater than those recommended by the Food and Drug Administration (FDA) have not been conducted. Case reports exist describing significant improvement in OC symptoms in two adult patients, one given sertraline 300 mg per day and the other citalopram 160 mg per day.[4,5] Both patients had received prior treatment with adequate trials of other SRIs, along with these particular medications at maximum recommended doses, without meaningful improvement. In contrast to SSRIs, clomipramine should generally not be given in doses greater than 250 mg per day owing to the risks of cardiotoxicity and seizures.

Intravenous clomipramine

Some patients have benefited from receiving clomipramine intravenously rather than by mouth. For example, a double-blind, placebo-controlled study of 14 daily intravenous (IV) infusions of clomipramine in adults with OCD refractory to or intolerant of oral clomipramine, and in many instances SSRIs, found the drug to be more effective than placebo.[6] Six of 29 patients randomized to IV clomipramine versus none of 25 patients given placebo were categorized as responders after the 14 infusions. Statistically significant improvement was found on some but not all measures of OC symptom severity. No serious adverse effects occurred. The authors hypothesized that the preferential efficacy of IV over oral clomipramine might be due to the greater bioavailability of the more serotonergic parent compound clomipramine compared with the more noradrenergic metabolite desmethyl-clomipramine, as a result of bypassing the first-pass hepatoenteric metabolism through the IV route. It has not been determined if patients who improve with IV clomipramine maintain their response when switched to oral medication. Liquid clomipramine for IV administration is not approved by the FDA for use in the USA, although it is available in many European countries and Canada. Further research on this treatment approach is in progress, including attempts to study IV versus oral pulse loading of clomipramine.[7]

Combination drug treatment strategies

Researchers have been pursuing two primary directions of combination drug treatment strategies for patients unimproved or only minimally improved following adequate trials of SRIs.[8,9] The first involves adding drugs that may further enhance serotonin (5-hydroxytryptamine, 5-HT) function to ongoing SRI administration. This approach has proved particularly effective in refractory major depressive disorder, where lithium augmentation of antidepressant treatment has been shown to be a useful intervention.[10] The second approach has been to add a dopamine (DA) receptor antagonist, such as a typical or atypical antipsychotic, to SRI therapy. The antipsychotic addition strategy has been largely based on phenomenological and genetic data linking some forms of OCD with chronic tic disorders such as Tourette's syndrome.[11]

SRIs plus drugs affecting 5-HT function

A number of drugs affecting 5-HT function, including tryptophan, fenfluramine, lithium, buspirone, clonazepam and pindolol, have been investigated for their potential to decrease OC symptoms when added to ongoing treatment with SRIs. The combination of clomipramine and an SSRI has also been studied.

Tryptophan

The addition of tryptophan, the amino acid precursor of 5-HT, to clomipramine treatment significantly improved OC symptoms in a single case study.[12] Others, however, have not found this approach to be useful,[13] and no controlled studies of this additional strategy have been published. Adverse neurological reactions resembling the 5-HT syndrome have been reported when tryptophan is used in combination with fluoxetine.[14] Furthermore, oral tryptophan is currently unavailable in the USA because of evidence linking some preparations with the eosinophilia myalgia syndrome.[15] Benefits of adding open-label tryptophan, up to 8 g per day, to an ongoing combination of SSRI and pindolol were reported by Blier and Bergeron in Canada (see below).[16]

Fenfluramine

Fenfluramine was recently withdrawn from the US market owing to concern that it contributed to the development of cardiac valvular disease.[17] It had previously been marketed for the treatment of obesity under the trade name Pondimin. Hollander et al reported that the addition of open-label D,L-fenfluramine, an indirect 5-HT agonist, to ongoing SRI treatment led to improvement in OC symptoms in six of seven patients.[18] In another report, two patients on clomipramine were observed to improve following the addition of D-fenfluramine, which is believed to have more specific effects on 5-HT transport and release than the racemic mixture, but which is also unavailable in the USA.[19] Some studies in laboratory animals have suggested that fenfluramine may be neurotoxic.[20] Furthermore, no controlled study of this combination treatment approach supporting its efficacy has been published.

Lithium

Lithium has been suggested to potentiate antidepressant-induced increases in 5-HT neurotransmission by enhancing presynaptic 5-HT release in some areas of the brain.[21] Although individual case reports suggested that lithium may further reduce OC symptoms when added to therapy with antidepressants,[22–24] including SRIs,[12,24–26] controlled studies have not substantiated these clinical observations.[27,28] Based on these results, the addition of lithium to ongoing SRI treatment of OCD does not appear to approach the rate or quality of response typically observed in antidepressant-refractory depression.[10] Clinical experience suggests that lithium augmentation of ongoing SRI therapy may be an option for patients who have primary major depressive disorder with secondary OC symptoms.

Buspirone

Buspirone is a 5-HT_{1A} receptor partial agonist and its chronic administration has been shown in preclinical studies to enhance 5-HT neurotransmission.[29] Results from two open-label studies of buspirone as an adjunct to fluoxetine treatment indicated that this approach led to a greater reduction in OC symptoms than did treatment with fluoxetine alone.[30,31] However, results from three double-blind, placebo-controlled studies of buspirone addition in adult OCD patients refractory to SRI monotherapy have not corroborated these initial reports.[32–34] Based on the authors' clinical experience, the addition of buspirone to SRI treatment can at times improve depressive symptoms in OCD patients with comorbid major depressive disorder.

In light of the efficacy of SRIs in OCD, presumably partly due to their ability to enhance central 5-HT neurotransmission, a better response to the controlled addition of lithium and buspirone might have been predicted. Both of these drugs have been shown to facilitate 5-HT function in the brain when given over time.[29,35] This neurochemical effect, however, may not be sufficient for achieving efficacy in the treatment of OCD. Blier and de Montigny have pointed out that the lack of response to lithium augmentation in OCD may be due to differential regional effects of lithium on 5-HT release in the central nervous system.[36] The same may be true for buspirone. For instance, preclinical studies have shown that lithium can enhance 5-HT release in the spinal cord,[37] hypothalamus,[38] and hippocampus,[39] whereas quantitative autoradiographic techniques have demonstrated high densities of 5-HT_{1A} receptors in the hippocampus, lateral septum, entorhinal cortex, and central amygdala.[40] In contrast, the cerebral cortex, caudate putamen, globus pallidus and substantia nigra, areas of the brain demonstrated to mediate some forms of OC phenomena, have not been found to be integrally involved in the mechanism of action of these two drugs.[40–42] Thus, although both agents may increase 5-HT neurotransmission in the brain, the activity may not be occurring in areas relevant to the treatment of OCD.

Clonazepam

Evidence from studies in laboratory animals and humans suggests that the benzodiazepine clonazepam may have effects on 5-HT function unlike those of other drugs in its class.[43] In a 4-week double-blind, placebo-controlled crossover study of clonazepam addition (3–4 mg per day) to ongoing fluoxetine or clomipramine, Pigott et al found significant improvement in one of three measures of OCD, but not the Y-BOCS.[44] The patients did show a significant reduction in ratings of anxiety. To our knowledge, this study has not been published beyond abstract form. In general, benzodiazepines may help secondary anxiety but are usually not effective for reducing the core symptoms of OCD.

Pindolol

The addition of pindolol to antidepressants has been reported to enhance or quicken response in adults with major depression in some[45,46] but not all studies.[47] Pindolol is hypothesized to act as a presynaptic 5-HT_{1A} antagonist, blocking somatodendritic 5-HT_{1A} autoreceptors on the cell bodies of 5-HT neurons in the midbrain raphe nuclei from the effects of acute increases in synaptic 5-HT induced by the antidepressant drug.[48] This action possibly antagonizes the usual resultant decrease in firing rate of the neuron and 5-HT release and thus hastens and facilitates 5-HT neurotransmission. In an open-label trial by Koran et al, pindolol 2.5 mg three times a day to 5.0 mg twice a day, for 2 weeks to 5 months, was added to ongoing SRI in eight adults with OCD who were minimally improved on their previous regimen.[49] One patient showed a complete resolution of OC symptoms within 4 days of pindolol addition, which was maintained during a 5-month follow-up. None of the other seven patients, however, had any significant improvement. In another open-label study, pindolol 2.5 mg three times a day for 4 weeks was added to ongoing SRI treatment in 13 patients minimally improved on SRI alone.[16] Four patients showed a meaningful improvement in OC symptoms as measured with the Y-BOCS. Of these four patients, three had comorbid major depression which improved markedly with pindolol addition. Overall, however, there was no significant group effect of pindolol addition on OC symptoms. To our knowledge, no controlled study of pindolol addition to SRIs in OCD has been published. These open-label reports suggest that this approach may be useful for the comorbid depressive symptoms of OCD but that it is unlikely to benefit the core OC symptoms for most patients.

Combining SRIs

No controlled study of the simultaneous administration of two SSRIs has been published in the treatment of OCD. A small open-label case series has described encouraging results with the coadministration of clomipramine and fluoxetine in adolescents with OCD.[50] Initially, six patients, mean age 14.8 years, were given clomipramine, mean dosage 92 mg per day, for a mean duration of 17.5 weeks. Three patients showed moderate improvement, whereas the other three were minimally improved on clomipramine alone. With combined clomipramine–

fluoxetine treatment, clinical global improvement was marked in five patients and moderate in one within weeks to months of adding fluoxetine. Optimal daily doses of clomipramine were 50 mg in four patients and 25 mg in two, and those of fluoxetine were 20 mg in four patients and 60 mg in two. The authors concluded that relatively low doses of a clomipramine–fluoxetine combination result in greater clinical global improvement, broader symptomatic relief, and fewer adverse effects in adolescents with OCD than with therapeutic doses of clomipramine alone. The beneficial effects of a clomipramine–fluoxetine combination have also been reported in three adult cases of severe OCD.[51] In a retrospective, open-label case series, seven children and young adults aged 9–23 received combined clomipramine–SSRI treatment with beneficial results.[52] None of the patients was able to tolerate high doses of either medication alone and all remained significantly impaired on monotherapy. Doses of clomipramine ranged from 25 mg to 100 mg daily in combination with different SSRIs. Two patients developed tachycardia and prolongation of the corrected QT interval on electrocardiography with the combined treatment. Because of the risk of SSRI-induced elevations of plasma levels of tricyclic antidepressants, including clomipramine, extreme caution should be used when giving these drugs concurrently. Because of clomipramine's potential to lower the seizure threshold and impede cardiac conduction, it is important to obtain clomipramine blood levels before and after the administration of an SSRI. Serial electrocardiograms should be obtained if this strategy is employed.

SRIs plus drugs affecting dopamine function

There has been no published controlled study of dopamine receptor antagonist monotherapy in the treatment of OCD as defined by the *Diagnostic and Statistical Manual of Mental Disorders*, 4th edition (DSM-IV).[53] In our clinical experience, DA receptor blockers are not effective when used alone for the treatment of OCD. However, these drugs remain the most effective treatment for tics, such as those typical of Tourette's syndrome.[54] In light of the phenomenologic, neurobiologic and genetic overlap between Tourette's syndrome and some forms of OCD,[55] the role of typical and atypical antipsychotic drugs as adjunctive treatments for SRI-refractory OCD has been explored.

Typical antipsychotic drugs

Pimozide

In an open-label case series, typical antipsychotics, primarily pimozide (6.5 mg per day), were added to ongoing treatment in 17 non-psychotic adult OCD patients unresponsive to fluvoxamine with or without lithium.[56] Nine of 17 patients were rated as 'much improved' or 'very much improved' on the CGI scale within 2–8 weeks of pimozide addition. Seven of eight patients with comorbid chronic tic disorder or schizotypal personality disorder were responders compared with only two of nine patients without this comorbidity.

Haloperidol

In a double-blind comparison with placebo, haloperidol (mean dose 6.2 mg per day) was significantly more effective when added to ongoing treatment in adult OCD patients unimproved on fluvoxamine alone.[57] Significant improvement was observed beginning 3 weeks after haloperidol addition. Eleven of 17 patients randomly assigned to receive haloperidol were rated as responders after 4 weeks of treatment compared with none of 17 patients who received placebo. Patients with a comorbid tic disorder showed a preferential response. Because of the small number of patients with comorbid schizotypal personality disorder in this investigation, it was not possible to make definitive conclusions about the usefulness of this approach for these patients. Based upon our clinical experience since completion of the study, we now typically begin haloperidol 0.25–0.5 mg per day, with subsequent increases every 4–7 days to a maximum of 2–4 mg per day, as clinically indicated. We have found that when this treatment strategy is effective, response will usually occur with lower doses of the DA receptor blocker than previously described, and usually within 2–4 weeks of addition to the SRI.

Atypical antipsychotic drugs

The atypical antipsychotic drugs, which modulate both DA and 5-HT function, and may be associated with lower risks of acute extrapyramidal side effects and chronic dyskinesias, have received increasing attention as potential treatments for SRI-refractory OCD.

Clozapine

The first atypical antipsychotic agent to be systematically evaluated in OCD was clozapine. The study was an open-label trial of clozapine monotherapy in 12 adults with refractory OCD.[58] Ten of 12 patients who entered the study completed the 10-week trial. Two patients dropped out prematurely due to sedation (100 mg per day for 3 weeks) and hypotension (125 mg per day for 2 weeks), respectively. The mean daily dose of clozapine in the 10 completers was 462.5 mg. Clozapine was not associated with any statistically significant improvement in OC or depressive symptoms or in a global measure of change. None of the patients met criteria for treatment response. To our knowledge, no report of clozapine addition to SRI treatment in OCD has appeared, and no controlled study has been conducted.

Risperidone

Clinical experience with risperidone in the treatment of SRI-refractory

OCD appears more promising than that with clozapine. To our knowledge, successful use of risperidone monotherapy in OCD has not been reported. Multiple open-label reports, however, have suggested that adding risperidone to ongoing SRI treatment in OCD patients minimally improved or unimproved on the SRI can be of significant benefit.[59–62] Interestingly, in contrast to the results from the study of haloperidol addition, it appears that patients with *and* without comorbid chronic tic disorders may respond to risperidone addition. The dosages of risperidone that appear helpful seem to be substantially lower (0.25 mg to 3 mg per day) than those generally employed for the treatment of psychotic symptoms in other patient populations. Furthermore, a decrease in OC symptoms is often observed within days of adding risperidone. Results from a double-blind, placebo-controlled study of risperidone addition to ongoing SRI treatment in adults with OCD are encouraging.[63] Fifty per cent of patients who were randomized to 6 weeks of risperidone (mean dose 2.2 mg per day) addition to ongoing SRI treatment were categorized as responders, compared with none of those who received placebo. There was no difference in treatment response between OCD patients with and without comorbid diagnoses of chronic tic disorders, and the drug was well tolerated.

Olanzapine

In an open-label study of olanzapine addition to ongoing SRI treatment in adults with OCD, ten patients who showed no response or partial improvement following an adequate SSRI trial were given olanzapine (mean dosage 7.3 mg per day) in conjunction with ongoing SRI for 8 weeks.[64] Four patients were categorized as responders, three as partial responders, and two as unchanged. The tenth patient discontinued olanzapine after only 3 weeks because of excessive sedation, in spite of apparent improvement in OC symptoms. Of the patients who completed the 8-week trial, one reported no side effects, seven reported sedation, and one experienced weight gain of 3.6 kg (8 lb).

To our knowledge, no report describing the use of the atypical antipsychotic quetiapine in OCD has appeared.

Bromocriptine

An open-label case series described a significant reduction in OC and depressive symptoms during chronic monotherapy with the DA receptor agonist bromocriptine (12.5–30 mg per day), in three of four adults with OCD and comorbid major depression.[65] Caution should be used with this approach because of the potential for the induction or exacerbation of tics. No controlled study of bromocriptine as monotherapy or an adjunctive treatment has been conducted in OCD.

SRIs plus drugs affecting other systems

Triiodothyronine

Sixteen adults with OCD who were partially improved on clomipramine received 4 weeks of triiodothyronine (liothyronine) 25 µg per day under double-blind conditions.[27] Thyroid hormone was not associated with any clinically meaningful change in OC or depressive symptoms.

Desipramine

Clomipramine has potent effects on both 5-HT and norepinephrine (noradrenaline) uptake. Based upon this mechanism of action, it has been suggested that effects on both neurochemical systems might be relevant to the drug's anti-OC efficacy. To address this question, Barr et al conducted a placebo-controlled study to investigate the addition of desipramine hydrochloride, a relatively selective norepinephrine reuptake inhibitor, to the regimen of 23 adults with OCD who were unimproved following 10 weeks of SSRI monotherapy.[66] No significant difference was found between desipramine and placebo, suggesting that clomipramine's anti-OC effect is largely mediated by its potent 5-HT, rather than norepinephrine, reuptake blocking properties.

Gabapentin

The neutral gamma-aminobutyric acid analog gabapentin was reported to further reduce OC symptoms when added in an open-label manner to ongoing treatment of five adults with OCD who were partially improved on fluoxetine 30–100 mg per day.[67] After 6 weeks, the mean daily dose of gabapentin was 2520 mg. Other than transient gastrointestinal side effects, the combination treatment was generally well tolerated. According to the report, all patients experienced marked subjective improvement in anxiety, OC symptoms, sleep and mood within 2 weeks of initiating gabapentin. These changes were corroborated by the evaluations of the clinical staff and supported by rating data when available. A double-blind, placebo-controlled study of this approach is reportedly currently under way by this research group.

A summary of the results of studies of combination drug treatment is given in Table 11.1.

Novel compounds

Inositol

The phosphatidylinositol cycle is the second messenger system for several neurotransmitters, including several subtypes of 5-HT receptors. Inositol (18 g per day), a simple polyol second messenger precursor, was administered to 15 adults with OCD in a double-blind, placebo-

Table 11.1   Double-blind, placebo-controlled drug studies in adults with treatment-refractory obsessive compulsive disorder.

May be effective:
- Intravenous clomipramine[a]
- Adding clonazepam[b]
- Adding haloperidol[c]
- Adding risperidone
- Inositol monotherapy[d]

Apparently ineffective:
- Adding lithium
- Adding buspirone
- Adding triiodothyronine (liothyronine)
- Adding desipramine

[a] Remains investigational in the USA.
[b] Only a small number of subjects studied, and improvement not evident on all OCD rating scales.
[c] Primarily in 'tic-related' OCD.
[d] A relatively small number of subjects were studied; remains investigational.

controlled crossover study (6 weeks each on drug and placebo).[68] For the 13 patients who completed the study, inositol resulted in a significant reduction in Y-BOCS scores compared with placebo, but no difference was shown between the two on the Hamilton depression or anxiety scales. No side effects occurred.

Tramadol

Tramadol is an opioid agonist which also inhibits the reuptake of 5-HT and norepinephrine (noradrenaline). Seven adults with SRI-refractory OCD entered a 6-week open-label study of tramadol.[69] Two patients discontinued the trial prematurely, the first during week 1 owing to nausea and exacerbation of trichotillomania, and the other during week 6 after experiencing a panic attack. The mean daily dose of tramadol for the six patients completing at least 2 weeks of treatment was 254 mg. After 6 weeks Y-BOCS scores were significantly reduced (by 26%), whereas Hamilton depression scores were not significantly different. The most frequent side effects were decreased appetite, insomnia, itching, sedation, dizziness and nausea. Three patients elected to continue treatment with the drug at the end of the trial.

Flutamide

Flutamide is a synthetic, non-steroidal, competitive antagonist of the androgen receptor. In an 8-week open-label study of flutamide, up to 750 mg per day, no significant improvement in OC, depressive or anxiety symptoms was found in eight adults with OCD.[70] The results from this study are consistent with two previous reports of the antiandrogen cyproterone acetate which showed lack of sustained effect[71] and no effect,[72] respectively, in adults with OCD.

Sumatriptan

Sumatriptan is a 5-HT$_{1D}$ agonist that is marketed for the treatment of migraine headache. In an open-label report, sumatriptan (100 mg per day) was given for 4 weeks to three adults with severe treatment-refractory OCD.[73] The drug reportedly led to a significant improvement in depressive symptoms and a modest reduction in OC symptoms. Upon discontinuation, symptoms returned in all three patients. No adverse effects were reported. As sumatriptan has been reported to penetrate the blood–brain barrier poorly, the mechanism of action of this drug in OCD remains unclear. To our knowledge, no controlled investigation of sumatriptan in OCD has been published.

Treatments warranting further study are listed in Table 11.2.

Other somatic treatments

Electroconvulsive therapy

In general, electroconvulsive therapy has not been considered an effective treatment for OCD. One report described a greater than 20% reduction in symptoms in a series of nine patients with treatment-refractory OCD without comorbid depression.[74] However, OC symptoms returned to pretreatment levels within 4 months.

Table 11.2   Promising treatments which may warrant controlled study for treatment-refractory obsessive compulsive disorder.

- Higher-dose SSRI monotherapy
- Adding pindolol
- Combined SSRI–clomipramine treatment
- Adding pimozide
- Adding olanzapine
- Bromocriptine monotherapy
- Adding gabapentin
- Tramadol monotherapy
- Sumatriptan monotherapy
- Repetitive transcranial magnetic stimulation
- Neurosurgery (gamma knife surgery)

Repetitive transcranial magnetic stimulation

Repetitive transcranial magnetic stimulation (rTMS) is a procedure in which a pulsatile high-intensity electromagnetic field is emitted from a coil placed against the scalp, resulting in focal electrical currents in the underlying cerebral cortex. Preliminary results from a controlled study by Greenberg et al suggest that a single application of rTMS to the right pre-frontal cortex produces a transient reduction of compulsive urges.[75] As seizures have occurred in some subjects receiving rTMS, the procedure is not without risk. Further study of rTMS as a potential treatment for OCD is continuing.

Neurosurgery

When non-surgical treatments have failed to improve OC symptoms signif-icantly in severely ill patients, at least partial relief can be obtained by some patients with neurosurgery. According to a review of this topic by Jenike, to be considered a candidate for a neurosurgical approach, patients must fail to improve following treatment with all available and appropriate psychotropic medications, as well as behavioral treatments.[76] Prior to being considered for surgery, each patient should have had ade-quate trials of clomipramine, fluoxetine, fluvoxamine, sertraline, paroxetine and a monoamine oxidase inhibitor, as well as augmentation of at least one of the above drugs for 1 month with at least two of the following: lithium, clonazepam and buspirone. If the patient has tics, a trial of aug-mentation with a low-dose neuroleptic should be performed. All patients must also have had an extended trial of behavior therapy consisting of exposure and response prevention. The illness must have been subject to intensive psychiatric treatment for such a lengthy period that it is, indeed, clearly refractory to standard treatment. In practice, most neurosurgical centers define this as a minimum of 5 years' duration. Various contraindi-cations also apply. In his review of the literature, Jenike concluded that, without further research, no definitive conclusions can be drawn as to which particular surgical procedure is the most effective among cingulo-tomy, anterior capsulotomy, limbic leukotomy and subcaudate tractotomy.

Results from thermocapsulotomy and gamma knife capsulotomy appear promising.[77] Preliminary pilot data from a controlled study of gamma knife surgery, where lesions are made in the anterior limb of the internal capsule as it passes up through the striatum from the dorso-medial and anterior thalamic nuclei to their projection sites in the orbito-medial frontal and cingulate cortices, have shown positive benefits.[78] In fact, efficacy has been demonstrated in 40–50% of the treatment-refractory patients receiving the active procedure with no significant acute or long-term side effects. Further double-blind studies to confirm efficacy and establish safety are needed.

Conclusion

This chapter has reviewed somatic interventions for patients with treatment-refractory OCD. Table 11.1 lists drug treatments that have been shown in double-blind, placebo-controlled studies to be either effective or ineffective for these patients. With regard to the negative studies listed in this table, it should be stated that such treatments may prove helpful for the individual patient. Treatments that appear promising, based upon open-label study results, and may warrant further systematic investigation, are listed in Table 11.2. Treatments that are likely to be ineffective, based upon open-label data, are listed in Table 11.3.

In addition to future controlled studies of these promising interventions, one area that warrants increased attention is the treatment of children and adolescents with refractory OCD. Preliminary reports suggest that combination drug treatments may be effective, but controlled studies of safety and efficacy are needed.[79,80]

Acknowledgments

The authors would like to thank Krista Guenin BA and Mrs Robbie Smith for their assistance in preparation of the manuscript. This work was supported, in part, by the Theodore and Vada Stanley Research Foundation (Dr McDougle), an Independent Investigator Award – Seaver Investigator from the National Alliance for Research on Schizophrenia and Depression (Dr McDougle), a Research Unit on Pediatric Psychopharmacology contract (N01MH70001) from the National Institute of Mental Health (Dr McDougle), and the State of Indiana Department of Mental Health.

Table 11.3 Treatments unlikely to be effective for treatment-refractory obsessive compulsive disorder.

- Adding tryptophan
- Adding fenfluramine
- Clozapine monotherapy
- Flutamide monotherapy
- Electroconvulsive therapy

References

1   McDougle CJ, Goodman WK, Leckman JF et al, The psychopharmacology of obsessive compulsive disorder: implications for treatment and pathogenesis, *Psychiatr Clin North Am* (1993) **16**:749–66.

2   Goodman WK, Price LH, Rasmussen SA et al, The Yale-Brown Obsessive Compulsive Scale (Y-BOCS): Part I. Development, use, and reliability, *Arch Gen Psychiatry* (1989) **46**:1006–11.

3   Goodman WK, Price LH, Rasmussen SA et al, The Yale-Brown Obsessive Compulsive Scale (Y-BOCS): Part II. Validity, *Arch Gen Psychiatry* (1989) **46**: 1012–16.

4   Byerly MJ, Goodman WK, Christensen R, High doses of sertraline for treatment-resistant obsessive-compulsive disorder, *Am J Psychiatry* (1996) **153**:1232–3.

5   Bejerot S, Bodlund O, Response to high doses of citalopram in treatment-resistant obsessive-compulsive disorder, *Acta Psych Scand* (1998) **98**:423–4.

6   Fallon BA, Liebowitz MR, Campeas R et al, Intravenous clomipramine for obsessive-compulsive disorder refractory to oral clomipramine: a placebo-controlled study, *Arch Gen Psychiatry* (1998) **55**:918–24.

7   Koran LM, Sallee FR, Pallanti S, Rapid benefit of intravenous pulse loading of clomipramine in obsessive-compulsive disorder, *Am J Psychiatry* (1997) **154**: 396–401.

8   McDougle CJ, Update on pharmacologic management of OCD: agents and augmentation, *J Clin Psychiatry* (1997) **58**(suppl. 12): 11–17.

9   Goodman WK, Ward HE, Murphy TK, Biologic approaches to treatment-refractory obsessive-compulsive disorder, *Psychiatr Ann* (1998) **28**:641–9.

10 Price LH, Heninger GR, Lithium in the treatment of mood disorders, *N Engl J Med* (1994) **331**:591–8.

11 McDougle CJ, Goodman WK, Price LH, Dopamine antagonists in tic-related and psychotic spectrum obsessive compulsive disorder, *J Clin Psychiatry* (1994) **55**(suppl. 3): 24–31.

12 Rasmussen SA, Lithium and tryptophan augmentation in clomipramine resistant obsessive-compulsive disorder, *Am J Psychiatry* (1984) **141**:1283–5.

13 Mattes J, A pilot study of combined trazodone and tryptophan in obsessive-compulsive disorder. *Int Clin Psychopharmacol* (1986) **1**:170–3.

14 Steiner W, Fontaine R, Toxic reaction following the combined administration of fluoxetine and L-tryptophan: five case reports. *Biol Psychiatry* (1986) **21**:1067–71.

15 Slutsker L, Hoesly FC, Miller L et al, Eosinophilia-myalgia syndrome associated with exposure to tryptophan from a single manufacturer, *JAMA* (1990) **264**: 213–17.

16 Blier P, Bergeron R, Sequential administration of augmentation strategies in treatment-resistant obsessive-compulsive disorder: preliminary findings, *Int Clin Psychopharmacol* (1996) **11**:37–44.

17 Connolly HM, Crary JL, McGoon MD et al, Valvular heart disease associated with fenfluramine-phentermine, *N Engl J Med* (1997) **337**:581–8.

18 Hollander E, DeCaria CM, Schneier FR et al, Fenfluramine augmentation of serotonin reuptake blockade antiobsessional treatment, *J Clin Psychiatry* (1990) **51**:119–23.

19   Judd FK, Chua P, Lynch C et al, Fenfluramine augmentation of clomipramine treatment of obsessive compulsive disorder, *Austr NZ J Psychiatry* (1991) **25**: 412–14.

20   Schuster C, Lewis M, Seiden L, Fenfluramine: neurotoxicity, *Psychopharm Bull* (1986) **22**:148–51.

21   De Montigny C, Enhancement of the 5-HT neurotransmission by antidepressant treatments, *J Physiol* (1981) **77**:455–61.

22   Stern TA, Jenike MA, Treatment of obsessive-compulsive disorder with lithium carbonate, *Psychosomatics* (1983) **24**:671–3.

23   Eisenberg J, Asnis G, Lithium as an adjunct treatment in obsessive-compulsive disorder, *Am J Psychiatry* (1985) **142**:663.

24   Golden RN, Morris JE, Sack DA, Combined lithium-tricyclic treatment of obsessive-compulsive disorder, *Biol Psychiatry* (1988) **23**:181–5.

25   Feder R, Lithium augmentation of clomipramine, *J Clin Psychiatry* (1988) **49**:458.

26   Ruegg RG, Evans DL, Comer WS, Lithium plus fluoxetine treatment of obsessive compulsive disorder, New Research Abstr. 92, 143rd Annual Meeting of the American Psychiatric Association, New York 1990; 81.

27   Pigott TA, Pato MT, L'Heureux F et al, A controlled comparison of adjuvant lithium carbonate or thyroid hormone in clomipramine-treated patients with obsessive-compulsive disorder, *J Clin Psychopharmacol* (1991) **11**:242–8.

28   McDougle CJ, Price LH, Goodman WK et al, A controlled trial of lithium augmentation in fluvoxamine-refractory obsessive compulsive disorder: lack of efficacy, *J Clin Psychopharmacol* (1991) **11**:175–84.

29   Blier P, de Montigny C, Chaput Y, A role for the serotonin system in the mechanism of action of antidepressant treatments: preclinical evidence, *J Clin Psychiatry* (1990) **51**(suppl. 4):14–20.

30   Markovitz PJ, Stagno SJ, Calabrese JR, Buspirone augmentation of fluoxetine in obsessive-compulsive disorder, *Am J Psychiatry* (1990) **147**:798–800.

31   Jenike MA, Baer L, Buttolph L, Buspirone augmentation of fluoxetine in patients with obsessive compulsive disorder, *Am J Clin Psychiatry* (1991) **52**:13–14.

32   Pigott TA, L'Heureux F, Hill JL et al, A double-blind study of adjuvant buspirone hydrochloride in clomipramine-treated patients with obsessive-compulsive disorder, *J Clin Psychopharmacol* (1992) **12**:11–18.

33   McDougle CJ, Goodman WK, Leckman JF et al, Limited therapeutic effect of addition of buspirone in fluvoxamine-refractory obsessive compulsive disorder, *Am J Psychiatry* (1993) **150**: 647–9.

34   Grady TA, Pigott TA, L'Heureux F et al, Double-blind study of adjuvant buspirone for fluoxetine-treated patients with obsessive-compulsive disorder, *Am J Psychiatry* (1993) **150**:819–21.

35   De Montigny C, Cournoyer G, Morissette R et al, Lithium carbonate addition in tricyclic antidepressant-resistant unipolar depression: correlations with the neurobiologic actions of tricyclic antidepressant drugs and lithium ion on the serotonin system, *Arch Gen Psychiatry* (1983) **40**: 1327–34.

36   Blier P, de Montigny C, Lack of efficacy of lithium augmentation in obsessive-compulsive disorder: the perspective of different regional effects of lithium on serotonin release in the central nervous system, *J Clin Psy-*

chopharmacol (1992) **12**:65–6.

37 Sangdee C, Franz DN, Lithium enhancement of 5-HT transmission induced by 5-HT precursors, *Biol Psychiatry* (1980) **15**:59–75.

38 Baptista TJ, Hernandez L, Burguera JL et al, Chronic lithium administration enhances serotonin release in the lateral hypothalamus but not in the hippocampus in rats: a microdialysis study, *J Neural Transm* (1990) **82**:31–41.

39 Treiser SL, Cascio CS, O'Donohue TL et al, Lithium increases serotonin release and decreases serotonin receptors in the hippocampus, *Science* (1981) **213**: 1529–31.

40 Radja F, Laporte AM, Daval G, Autoradiography of serotonin receptor subtypes in the central nervous system, *Neurochem Int* (1991) **18**:1–15.

41 Friedman E, Hoau-Yan W, Effect of chronic lithium treatment of 5-hydroxytryptamine autoreceptors and release of 5[^{3}H]hydroxytryptamine from rat brain cortical, hippocampal, and hypothalamic slices, *J Neurochem* (1988) **50**:195–201.

42 Katz RJ, Chase TN, Irwin JK, Evoked release of norepinephrine and serotonin from brain slices: inhibition by lithium, *Science* (1968) **162**:466–7.

43 Wagner HR, Reches A, Yablonskaya E et al, Clonazepam-induced up-regulation of serotonin-1 and serotonin-2 binding sites in rat frontal cortex, *Adv Neurol* (1986) **43**:645–51.

44 Pigott TA, L'Heureux FL, Rubenstein CS, A controlled trial of clonazepam augmentation in OCD patients treated with clomipramine or fluoxetine, New Research Abstr. 144, 145th Annual Meeting of the American Psychiatric Association, Washington, DC, 1992; 82.

45 Artigas F, Romero L, de Montigny C et al, Acceleration of the effect of selected antidepressant drugs in major depression by 5-HT1A antagonists, *Trends Neurosci* (1996) **19**:378–83.

46 Blier P, Bergeron R, Effectiveness of pindolol with selected antidepressant drugs in the treatment of major depression, *J Clin Psychopharmacol* (1995) **15**:217–22.

47 Berman RM, Darnell AM, Miller HL et al, Effect of pindolol in hastening response to fluoxetine in the treatment of major depression: a double-blind, placebo-controlled trial, *Am J Psychiatry* (1997) **154**:37–43.

48 Artigas F, Perez V, Alvarez E, Pindolol induces a rapid improvement of depressed patients treated with serotonin reuptake inhibitors, *Arch Gen Psychiatry* (1994) **51**:248–51.

49 Koran LM, Mueller K, Maloney A, Will pindolol augment the response to a serotonin reuptake inhibitor in obsessive-compulsive disorder? *J Clin Psychopharmacol* (1996) **16**:253–4.

50 Simeon JG, Thatte S, Wiggins D, Treatment of adolescent obsessive-compulsive disorder with a clomipramine-fluoxetine combination, *Psychopharm Bull* (1990) **26**:285–90.

51 Browne M, Horn E, Jones TT, The benefits of clomipramine-fluoxetine combination in obsessive compulsive disorder, *Can J Psychiatry* (1993) **38**:242–3.

52 Figueroa Y, Rosenberg DR, Birmaher B et al, Combination treatment with clomipramine and selective serotonin reuptake inhibitors for obsessive-compulsive disorder in children and adolescents, *J Child Adolesc Psych* (1998) **8**:61–7.

53 American Psychiatric Association,

Diagnostic and Statistical Manual of Mental Disorders, 4th edn (American Psychiatric Association: Washington, DC, 1994).

54 Leckman JF, Pauls DL, Cohen DJ, Tic disorders. In: Bloom FE, Kupfer DJ, eds, *Psychopharmacology: The Fourth Generation of Progress* (Raven Press: New York, 1995) 1665–74.

55 Goodman WK, McDougle CJ, Price LH et al, Beyond the serotonin hypothesis: a role for dopamine in some forms of obsessive compulsive disorder? *J Clin Psychiatry* (1990) **51**(suppl.): 36–43.

56 McDougle CJ, Goodman WK, Price LH, Neuroleptic addition in fluvoxamine-refractory obsessive-compulsive disorder, *Am J Psychiatry* (1990) **147**:652–4.

57 McDougle CJ, Goodman WK, Leckman JF et al, Haloperidol addition in fluvoxamine-refractory obsessive compulsive disorder: a double-blind, placebo-controlled study in patients with and without tics, *Arch Gen Psychiatry* (1994) **51**:302–8.

58 McDougle CJ, Barr LC, Goodman WK et al, Lack of efficacy of clozapine monotherapy in refractory obsessive compulsive disorder. *Am J Psychiatry* (1995) **152**: 1812–14.

59 Jacobsen FM, Risperidone in the treatment of affective illness and obsessive compulsive disorder, *J Clin Psychiatry* (1995) **56**:423–9.

60 McDougle CJ, Fleischmann RL, Epperson CN et al, Risperidone addition in fluvoxamine-refractory obsessive compulsive disorder: three cases, *J Clin Psychiatry* (1995) **56**:526–8.

61 Saxena S, Wang D, Bystritsky A et al, Risperidone augmentation of SRI treatment for refractory obsessive-compulsive disorder, *J Clin Psychiatry* (1996) **57**:303–6.

62 Stein DJ, Bouwer C, Hawkridge S et al, Risperidone augmentation of serotonin reuptake inhibitors in obsessive-compulsive and related disorders, *J Clin Psychiatry* (1997) **58**:119–22.

63 McDougle CJ, Epperson CN, Pelton GH et al, A double-blind, placebo-controlled study of risperidone addition in serotonin reuptake inhibitor-refractory obsessive-compulsive disorder, *Arch Gen Psychiatry* (2000) **57**:794–801.

64 Weiss EL, Potenza MN, McDougle CJ et al, Olanzapine addition in obsessive-compulsive disorder refractory to selective serotonin reuptake inhibitors: an open-label case series, *J Clin Psychiatry* (1999) **60**:524–7.

65 Ceccherini-Nelli A, Guazzelli M, Treatment of refractory OCD with the dopamine agonist bromocriptine, *J Clin Psychiatry* (1994) **55**:415–16.

66 Barr LC, Goodman WK, Anand A et al, Addition of desipramine to serotonin reuptake inhibitors in treatment-resistant obsessive compulsive disorder, *Am J Psychiatry* (1997) **154**:1293–5.

67 Cora-Locatelli G, Greenberg BD, Martin J et al, Gabapentin augmentation for fluoxetine-treated patients with obsessive-compulsive disorder, *J Clin Psychiatry* (1998) **59**:480–1.

68 Fux M, Levine J, Aviv A et al, Inositol treatment of obsessive-compulsive disorder, *Am J Psychiatry* (1996) **153**:1219–21.

69 Shapira NA, Keck PE, Goldsmith TD et al, Open-label pilot study of tramadol hydrochloride in treatment-refractory obsessive-compulsive disorder, *Depress Anx* (1997) **6**:170–3.

70 Altemus M, Greenberg BD, Keuler D et al, Open trial of flutamide for treatment of obsessive-

compulsive disorder, *J Clin Psychiatry* (1999) **60**:442–5.

71 Casas M, Alvarez E, Duro P et al, Antiandrogenic treatment of obsessive-compulsive neurosis, *Acta Psych Scand* (1986) **73**: 221–2.

72 Feldman JD, Noshirvani H, Chu C, Improvement in female patients with severe obsessions and/or compulsions treated with cyproterone acetate, *Acta Psych Scand* (1988) **78**:254.

73 Stern L, Zohar J, Cohen R et al, Treatment of severe, drug resistant obsessive compulsive disorder with the 5HT1D agonist sumatriptan, *Eur Neuropsychopharmacol* (1998) **8**:325–8.

74 Khanna S, Gangadhar BN, Sinha V et al, Electroconvulsive therapy in obsessive-compulsive disorder, *Convuls Ther* (1988) **4**: 314–20.

75 Greenberg BD, George MS, Martin DJ et al, Effect of prefrontal repetitive transcranial magnetic stimulation in obsessive compulsive disorder: a preliminary study, *Am J Psychiatry* (1997) **154**: 687–9.

76 Jenike MA, Neurosurgical treatment of obsessive-compulsive disorder, *Br J Psychiatry* (1998) **173**(suppl. 35):79–90.

77 Lippitz BE, Mindus P, Meyerson BA et al, Lesion topography and outcome after thermocapsulotomy or gamma knife capsulotomy for obsessive-compulsive disorder: relevance of the right hemisphere, *Neurosurgery* (1999) **44**:452–60.

78 Rasmussen SA, Eisen JL, Treatment strategies for chronic and refractory obsessive-compulsive disorder, *J Clin Psychiatry* (1997) **58**(suppl. 13):9–13.

79 Leonard HL, Topol D, Bukstein O et al, Clonazepam as an augmenting agent in the treatment of childhood-onset obsessive compulsive disorder, *J Am Acad Child Adolesc Psych* (1994) **33**: 792–4.

80 Fitzgerald KD, Stewart CM, Tawile V et al, Risperidone augmentation of serotonin reuptake inhibitor treatment of pediatric obsessive compulsive disorder, *J Child Adolesc Psychopharmacol* (1999) **9**:115–23.

12

Obsessive compulsive disorder in children and adolescents

Martine F Flament and David Cohen

Despite early descriptions of typical cases of obsessive compulsive disorder (OCD) in children, it was believed until recently that the disorder was rare in young people. Ritualistic and compulsive-like activity was considered to be part of the normal development of the behavioural repertoire. The first systematic evidence of obsessive compulsive symptoms occurring at an early age came from retrospective studies with adult OCD patients, suggesting that in 30% to 50% their disorder began during childhood or adolescence.[1,2] Epidemiological data subsequently showed that OCD was far more prevalent among adolescents than previously thought. A number of systematic studies conducted on children and adolescents with OCD, both in clinical settings and in the community, have greatly increased our knowledge of the disorder in its early stage. They have shown that, in contrast to other forms of psychopathology, the specific features of OCD are essentially identical in children, adolescents and adults. With a tremendous growth of interest and research on childhood-onset OCD, significant advances have occurred regarding phenomenology, epidemiology, genetics, neurophysiology, pathogenesis and treatment of the disorder.

Clinical features

The clinical presentation of OCD during childhood and adolescent years has been documented in various countries and various cultures, with large clinical series reported from the USA,[3] Japan,[4] India,[5] Israel,[6] Denmark[7] and Spain.[8] In clinical samples, as in community-based samples,[9] obsessions most commonly concern fear of dirt or germs, harm coming to self or a loved one, symmetry or scrupulous religiosity, and the most frequent presenting rituals include washing, repeating, checking, touching, ordering, counting and hoarding. Typically, children and adolescents with OCD experience multiple obsessions and compulsions, whose nature may change over time. Generally, compulsions are carried out to dispel anxiety and/or in response to an obsession (e.g. to ward off harm to someone). Some of the obsessions and rituals involve an internal sense that 'it does not feel right' until the thought or action is completed. No significant age-related trends have been found for either the number or the type of symptoms, except that patients with very early onset tend to have more compulsions than obsessions.[10]

Onset of OCD in children and adolescents may be acute or gradual. Reports of the mean age at onset in referred subjects have ranged from 9.0 years[11] to 11.6 years,[4] and it was 12.8 years in a community study.[9] In community-based samples of adolescents with OCD there are approximately equal numbers of boys and girls, whereas in most studies of referred children and adolescents boys outnumber girls 2 : 1. Overrepresentation of boys in clinical samples may reflect a greater severity of the disorder and an earlier age of onset than in girls.[12]

It has been consistently observed, in both clinical and community studies, that childhood OCD is frequently accompanied by other symptoms, with an overall lifetime comorbidity as high as 75%.[13] Mood and anxiety disorders are the most common comorbid conditions, with prevalence ranging across studies from 20% to 73%,[14,15] and from 26% to 70%,[3,15] respectively. Anorexia nervosa has been reported in 8% of OCD adolescents;[8] conversely, OCD has been found in 3% to 66% of girls with anorexia nervosa.[16] Of particular clinical importance is the high rate of comorbid tic disorders, including Tourette's disorder, which have been reported in 17% to 40% of referred OCD patients,[8,15] and in 25% of a community-derived sample.[17]

Although findings regarding the significance of potential subtypes of OCD remain to be confirmed, some authors have suggested that the distinction between 'tic-related OCD' and 'non-tic-related OCD', or between early (prepubertal) and later (pubertal) onset, may be a useful one.[18]

Epidemiology

In adolescents, epidemiological studies using strict diagnostic criteria and structured clinical interviews have been conducted in several parts of the world, estimating the prevalence of OCD between 1% and 4%.[19] In the largest study, conducted in a US population of 5596 high-school students,[9] the current prevalence of OCD in adolescents was 1 (± 0.5)%, and its lifetime prevalence 1.9 (± 0.7)%. The study showed that the disorder was clearly underdiagnosed and undertreated in this age group: none of the cases identified had been previously diagnosed, and only 20% had ever been treated for comorbid psychological problems. In a later study examining 562 consecutive inductees into the Israeli army, the point prevalence of OCD was 3.6 (± 0.7)%.[17] Of note was the high proportion of subjects with obsessions only (50%), potentially less disruptive of everyday functioning. If the prevalence of OCD was estimated excluding individuals who only had obsessions, the point prevalence dropped to 1.8%. In two longitudinal studies following cohorts of children in the community up to the age of 18 years, one from the USA found a lifetime prevalence for OCD of 2.1%,[20] and the other from New Zealand an overall 1-year prevalence of 4%, but only 1.2% when subjects with obsessions only were excluded.[21] Thus, it appears that OCD might be as frequent in adolescents as it is in adults.

There has been no community study on the prevalence of OCD during childhood, but estimates of the frequency of OCD in clinical samples of children range from 1.3% to 5%.[18] They suggest that many youngsters with OCD still do not come to clinical attention.

Pathogenesis

Although a variety of biological causes for OCD have been proposed since 1860,[22] modern neurobiological theories began with clinical studies showing that clomipramine and other serotonin reuptake inhibitors had a unique efficacy in treating OCD. In children and adolescents, a few studies have provided evidence of the involvement of the serotonergic system in the pathophysiology of the disorder: there have been reports of decreased density of the platelet serotonin transporter in children and adolescents with OCD, but not in those with Tourette's disorder,[23,24] and another study showed an increase in central serotonin turnover in children and adolescents with OCD, compared with children and adolescents with disruptive behaviour disorder.[25]

Several family studies have shown that OCD is much more frequent among relatives of individuals with the disorder than would be expected from estimated occurrence rates for the general population. Lenane et al, interviewing first-degree relatives of 46 children and adolescents with OCD, found that 25% of the fathers and 9% of the mothers had OCD, and that the age-corrected risk for OCD and subthreshold OCD combined for all first-degree relatives was 35%.[26] Pauls et al reported that the prevalence rates of OCD and tic disorders were significantly greater among the first-degree relatives of 100 probands with OCD (10.3% and 4.6%, respectively) than among relatives of psychiatrically unaffected subjects (1.9% and 1.0%); interestingly, there was a two-fold increased risk for OCD and a four-fold increased risk for subthreshold OCD in relatives of probands with early onset (≤18 years) of OCD, compared with those with a later onset.[27]

Data from neuroimaging studies have brought definite evidence of morphological and/or functional abnormalities associated with at least some forms of OCD. One computerized tomography study found significantly smaller caudate volumes in young men with childhood-onset OCD compared with controls,[28] and one magnetic resonance morphologic study reported that children with OCD had significantly larger anterior cingulate gyri than did controls.[29] Studies using functional neuroimaging have tended to demonstrate metabolic abnormalities in the circuits involving orbitofrontal/cingulate cortex and the basal ganglia.[30] Furthermore, five of seven studies comparing brain functioning in OCD patients before and after successful pharmacological or psychological therapy demonstrated reduction of the hypermetabolism of the frontal lobes following treatment. One of these studies was conducted before and after pharmacological treatment in childhood-onset OCD patients.[31,32]

Autoimmune factors have also been implicated in the possible pathogenesis of OCD. Two independent groups of investigators demonstrated a strong association between acute-onset OCD and Sydenham's chorea, a childhood movement disorder associated with rheumatic fever, which is thought to result from an antineuronal antibody-mediated response to group A β-haemolytic streptococcus (GABHS) directed at portions of the basal ganglia, in genetically vulnerable individuals.[33,34] Even in the absence of the neurological symptoms of Sydenham's chorea, post-streptococcal cases of childhood-onset OCD, tics and/or other neuropsychiatric symptoms have been described under the acronym of PANDAS (Paediatric Autoimmune Neuropsychiatric Disorders Associated with Streptococcal infections).[35] These findings of a probable autoimmune basis for OCD led Swedo and colleagues to successfully apply immunomodulatory treatments in children with severe, infection-triggered exacerbations of OCD or tic disorders.[36] However, the first double-blind attempt to demonstrate the efficacy of penicillin prophylaxis in preventing tic or obsessive compulsive symptoms exacerbation in PANDAS failed to do so, because of inability to achieve an acceptable level of streptococcal prophylaxis.[37]

Treatment

The treatment of OCD has changed dramatically since the 1980s, with two approaches systematically assessed and empirically shown to ameliorate the core symptoms of the disorder in children and adolescents: pharmacological treatment with agents that are potent serotonin reuptake inhibitors, and specific cognitive behavioural treatment.

Psychopharmacological treatment

Several randomized, controlled clinical trials and some additional open studies have been conducted in children and adolescents with OCD, demonstrating (like many similar studies in adult patients) the selective and unique efficacy of serotonin reuptake inhibitors in the short-term treatment of the disorder. The design and main results of these studies are summarized in Table 12.1.

Table 12.1 Pharmacological treatment studies of OCD in children and adolescents.

Study (year)	N (age) Duration of treatment	Drug (daily dose) Study design	Improvement on active drug across measures (%)
Flament et al (1985)[38]	19 (6–18 yr) 5 weeks	Clomipramine (mean: 141 mg) vs placebo	22–44
Leonard et al (1989)[40]	47 (7–19 yr) 5 weeks	Clomipramine (mean:150 mg) vs desipramine	19–29
DeVeaugh-Geiss et al (1992)[39]	60 (10–17 yr) 8 weeks	Clomipramine (75–200 mg) vs placebo	34–37
Riddle et al (1992)[42]	14 (8–15 yr) 8 weeks	Fluoxetine (20 mg) vs placebo	33–44
Apter et al (1994)[43]	14 (13–18 yr) 8 weeks	Fluvoxamine (100–300 mg) open study	28
Thomsen (1997)[44]	23 (9–18 yr) 10 weeks	Citalopram (mean: 37 mg) open study	20–29
March et al (1998)[46]	187 (6–17 yr) 12 weeks	Sertraline (mean: 167 mg) vs placebo	21–28
Rosenberg et al (1999)[45]	20 (8–17 yr) 12 weeks	Paroxetine (mean: 41 mg) open study	28

Clomipramine was the first known antiobsessional agent. Its efficacy in children and adolescents with OCD has been demonstrated in two placebo-controlled studies,[38,39] and in one study comparing it with desipramine.[40] Moderate or marked improvement with clomipramine (at doses ranging from 75 mg to 200 mg per day) was apparent by 5 weeks of treatment in about 75% of subjects; this was independent of the presence of depressive symptoms at baseline. In one study, improvement of obsessive compulsive symptoms was closely correlated with pretreatment platelet serotonin concentration, and with the decrease of this measure during treatment.[41] Fluoxetine was investigated in a small placebo-controlled study,[42] and open label trials have been published for fluvoxamine,[43] citalopram,[44] and paroxetine.[45] The largest controlled study completed to date is a multicentre placebo-controlled trial of sertraline, in which significant differences between sertraline and placebo emerged at week 3 and persisted for the duration of the study.[46] The degree of symptomatic improvement with the selective serotonin reuptake inhibitors (SSRIs) is comparable to that observed in previous trials with clomipramine (Table 12.1).

The secondary effects of clomipramine include dry mouth, somnolence, dizziness, tremor, headache, constipation, stomach discomfort, sweating, insomnia, possible tachycardia and prolongation of the QT interval on electrocardiography (ECG); baseline and periodic ECG monitoring is recommended.[18] Published studies suggest that the SSRIs are safe and well tolerated in children and adolescents. Although there are differences between these drugs, the most commonly described side effects include nausea, headache, tremor, gastrointestinal complaints, drowsiness, insomnia, akathisia, disinhibition, agitation and hypomania. Systematic dose response data are not available for children, but side effects generally appear dose-dependent. It is therefore recommended to start an SSRI with a low dosage that is increased slowly up to the minimum daily dose found effective in adult patients (fluoxetine 20 mg, sertraline 50 mg, paroxetine 40 mg, citalopram 20 mg; no fixed-doses studies for fluvoxamine), although much higher doses have been used in published studies (Table 12.1).

For children and adolescents with OCD and comorbid tic disorder, SSRIs alone might have little antiobsessional effect, and there are reports suggesting that these agents, especially at higher doses, may exacerbate or even induce tics in some patients.[13] In such cases, the efficacy of a combined treatment with an SSRI and a dopamine antagonist has been demonstrated in adults, but still needs to be confirmed in younger patients.

The optimal duration of maintenance treatment is unclear, since relapses are frequent when medication is discontinued.[47] Antiobsessional medication should be maintained for at least 12–18 months after a satisfactory clinical response has been obtained. Once the decision is made to attempt reduction or discontinuation, the tapering should be gradual.

Cognitive behavioural treatment

Cognitive behavioural treatment (CBT) is regarded as the psychological treatment of choice for children and adolescents with OCD. In contrast to medication, where relapse is common when treatment is withdrawn, CBT has been shown to be a more durable treatment, although booster sessions may be required from time to time. Treatment generally involves a three-stage approach, consisting of information gathering, therapist-assisted graded exposure with response prevention, and homework assignments.[48] Interventions for children with predominantly internalizing symptoms also include relaxation and cognitive training. The family needs to be involved in the treatment to a varying extent according to individual situations. This therapy usually involves 13–20 weekly individual or family sessions and homework assignments. Partial or non-responders may require more frequent visits and therapist-assisted training at home.

Three open studies (Table 12.2) have shown beneficial effects of CBT, alone or in combination with pharmacotherapy, in groups of 14–15 children and adolescents with OCD: following treatment, symptoms were relieved entirely or reduced to a mildly incapacitating level in 50% to 86% of cases.[49–51] In a randomized trial comparing CBT and clomipramine,[52] CBT produced stronger therapeutic changes than clomipramine after 12 weeks, and, after another 12 weeks, five of the nine initial non-responders showed significant changes with a combination of both treatment regimens.

Other therapeutic approaches

Although some uncontrolled case studies have found psychodynamic psychotherapy useful in treating juvenile OCD,[53,54] the effectiveness of psychotherapy alone – apart from exposure techniques – on obsessive and compulsive symptoms has yet to be systematically explored. Nevertheless, traditional psychotherapeutic approaches may help children and adolescents address intrapsychic conflicts that affect or result from their illness.

Family psychopathology is neither necessary nor sufficient for the onset of OCD. Nonetheless, families affect and are affected by the disorder. Work with families on how to manage the child's symptom, cope with the stress and family disruption that often accompanies OCD, and participate effectively in behavioural or pharmacological treatment, is essential.[55] Family support groups and patient advocacy groups, now available in many countries, can also provide valuable help and support.

In cases of severe OCD, there is empirical evidence that milieu therapy in inpatient settings may be a useful resource.[49,53]

Table 12.2 Cognitive behavioural treatment ('CBT') studies of OCD in children and adolescents.

Study (year)	N (age) Duration of treatment	Study design	Short-term improvement	Long-term improvement
Bolton et al (1983)[49]	15 (12–18 yr) 1–48 months	Open trial CBT ± drug or other treatment	7 asymptomatic 6 much improved	9 months to 4 years: 11/14 improved
March et al (1994)[50]	15 (8–18 yr) 22 weeks	Open trial CBT ± drug or other treatment	6 asymptomatic 3 much improved	18 months: 9/15 improved
Franklin et al (1998)[51]	14 (10–17 yr) 1–4 months	Open trial CBT ± drug or other treatment	12 responders (≥50% decrease in OC symptoms)	9 months: 10/12 improved
De Haan et al (1998)[52]	22 (8–18 yr) 12 weeks	Randomised trial CBT ($n=12$) vs clomipramine ($n=10$)	8/12 responders (≥30% decrease in OC symptoms) on CBT vs 5/10 responders on clomipramine ($p < 0.05$)	Not reported

Course and outcome

Several retrospective and prospective follow-up studies have demonstrated the continuity of the diagnosis of OCD from childhood to adulthood: when subjects are still symptomatic, the main diagnosis is almost invariably OCD, although comorbid disorders, especially mood and/or anxiety disorders, are frequent; evolution towards psychosis is rare.[12] The spontaneous course is most often marked by a waxing and waning severity of the disorder, whereas remissions under treatment may be followed by relapses, even after long periods.

In the earliest follow-up studies, when no specific treatment was available, recovery rate in early adulthood ranged from 13%[56] to 28%.[9] By the time patients had access to specific treatments with SSRIs and/or CBT, recovery rates increased to 57–65%,[57–59] although in some studies many of the subjects symptom-free at follow-up were still taking medication.

Studies on the natural course of OCD and on the clinical response to treatment have attempted to identify demographic or clinical features that may influence outcome or course of illness – with mainly negative or inconsistent results.[12] Except for one short-term pharmacological study, in which male subjects responded significantly better than did female subjects,[38] the initial treatment response could not be predicted by sex, age of onset, duration or severity of illness, or type of symptoms. In a prospective follow-up study, over 2–7 years, a poorer long-term outcome was predicted by a higher obsessive compulsive symptom score after the first 5 weeks of pharmacotherapy (but not at baseline), and by the presence of a lifetime history of tic disorder or of a parental Axis I psychiatric diagnosis.[57]

Conclusion

Obsessive compulsive disorder is much more frequent in children and adolescents than previously thought. Youths with OCD suffer from a wide range of symptoms, including both obsessions and compulsions, that may change over time, but all longitudinal studies clearly demonstrate the continuity of the disorder from childhood to adulthood. Short-term and longer follow-up studies gave definite evidence that two types of treatment intervention can markedly improve the core symptoms of the disorder, and significantly reduce impairment from the condition. Cognitive behavioural treatment may be the initial treatment of choice in milder cases without significant comorbidity, whereas severity of obsessive compulsive symptoms, presence of comorbid conditions, or insufficient cognitive or emotional ability to cooperate in CBT, are indications for pharmacological treatment with a serotonin reuptake inhibitor. The combination treatment may be more effective than either alone, and CBT may reduce the relapse rate in patients withdrawn from medication.

Although the currently available treatments may not be curative, most children and adolescents given a correct diagnosis and an individually targeted treatment may be substantially helped to resume a normal developmental trajectory. However, more research is needed into the basic neurobiological mechanisms in OCD, to improve understanding and long-term outcome of what may prove to be an heterogeneous disorder.

References

1 Black A, The natural history of obsessional neurosis. In: Beech HR, ed., *Obsessional States* (Methuen: London, 1974)

2 Rasmussen SA, Eisen JL, Epidemiology of obsessive compulsive disorder, *J Clin Psychiatry* (1990) **51**(2 suppl.):10–13.

3 Swedo SE, Rapoport JL, Leonard H, Lenane M, Cheslow D, Obsessive-compulsive disorder in children and adolescents. Clinical phenomenology of 70 consecutive cases, *Arch Gen Psychiatry* (1989) **46**:335–40.

4 Honjo S, Hirano C, Murase S et al, Obsessive-compulsive symptoms in childhood and adolescence, *Acta Psychiatr Scand* (1989) **80**:83–91.

5 Khanna S, Srinath S, Childhood obsessive compulsive disorder. I. Psychopathology, *Psychopathology* (1989) **32**:47–54.

6 Apter A, Tyano S, Obsessive compulsive disorders in adolescence, *J Adolesc* (1988) **11**: 183–94.

7 Thomsen PH, Obsessive-compulsive symptoms in children and adolescents. A phenomenological analysis of 61 Danish cases, *Psychopathology* (1991) **24**:12–18.

8 Toro J, Cervera M, Osjeo E, Salamero M, Obsessive-compulsive disorder in childhood and adolescence: a clinical study, *J*

   Child Psychol Psychiat (1992) **33**:1025–37.

9 Flament MF, Whitaker A, Rapoport JL et al, Obsessive compulsive disorder in adolescence: an epidemiological study, *J Am Acad Child Adolesc Psychiatry* (1988) **27**:764–71.

10 Rettew DC, Swedo SE, Leonard HL, Lenane M, Rapoport JL, Obsessions and compulsions across time in 79 children and adolescents with obsessive-compulsive disorder, *J Am Acad Child Adolesc Psych* (1992) **31**: 1050–56.

11 Riddle MA, Scahill L, King R et al, Obsessive compulsive disorder in children and adolescents: phenomenology and family history, *J Am Acad Child Adolesc Psych* (1990) **29**:766–72.

12 Flament MF, Obsessive-compulsive disorder. In: Steinhausen HC, Verhulst F, eds *Risks and Outcomes in Developmental Psychopathology* (Oxford University Press: Oxford, 1999)

13 Flament MF, Cohen D, Child and adolescent obsessive compulsive disorder. In: Maj M, Sartorius N, eds, *Obsessive-compulsive Disorder. WPA Series Evidence and Experience in Psychiatry Vol. 4* (John Wiley & Sons Chichester, 2000; 147–83).

14 Flament MF, Koby E, Rapoport JL

et al, Childhood obsessive-compulsive disorder: a prospective follow-up study, *J Child Psychol Psychiat* (1990) **31**:363–80.

15 Geller DA, Biederman J, Griffin S, Jones J, Lefkowitz TD, Comorbidity of obsessive-compulsive disorder with disruptive behavior disorders, *J Am Acad Child Adolesc Psych* (1996) **35**:1637–46.

16 Godart N, Flament MF, Jeammet P, Lecrubier Y, Eating disorders and anxiety disorders: comorbidity and chronology of appearance, *Eur Psychiatry* (2000) **15**:38–45.

17 Zohar AH, Ratzosin G, Pauls DL et al, An epidemiological study of obsessive-compulsive disorder and related disorders in Israeli adolescents, *J Am Acad Child Adolesc Psych* (1992) **31**: 1057–61.

18 American Academy of Child and Adolescent Psychiatry, Practice parameters for the assessment and treatment of children and adolescents with obsessive-compulsive disorder, *J Am Acad Child Adolesc Psych* (1998) **37**(suppl 10):27–45S.

19 Flament MF, Chabane N, Obsessive-compulsive disorder and tics in children and adolescents. In: Gelder M, Lopez-Ibor JJ, Andreasen NC, eds, The *New Oxford Textbook of Psychiatry*, (Oxford University Press: Oxford, 2000; 1771–81).

20 Reinherz HZ, Giaconia RM, Lefkowitz ES, Pakiz B, Frost AK, Prevalence of psychiatric disorders in a community population of older adolescents, *J Am Acad Child Adolesc Psych* (1993) **32**:369–77.

21 Douglass HM, Moffitt TE, Dar R, McGee R, Silva P, Obsessive-compulsive disorder in a birth cohort of 18-year-olds: prevalence and predictors, *J Am Acad Child Adolesc Psych* (1995) **34**: 1424–31.

22 Rapoport JL, The neurobiology of obsessive compulsive disorder, *JAMA* (1989) **260**:2888–90.

23 Weizman A, Mandel A, Barber Y et al, Decreased platelet imipramine binding in Tourette syndrome children with obsessive-compulsive disorder, *Biol Psychiatry* (1992) **31**:705–11.

24 Sallee FR, Richman H, Beach K et al, Platelet serotonin transporter in children and adolescents with obsessive-compulsive disorder or Tourette's syndrome, *J Am Acad Child Adolesc Psych* (1996) **35**: 1647–56.

25 Zahn TP, Kruesi MJP, Swedo SE et al, Autonomic activity in relation to cerebrospinal fluid neurochemistry in obsessive and disruptive children and adolescents, *Psychophysiology* (1992) **33**:731–9.

26 Lenane MC, Swedo SE, Leonard H et al, Psychiatric disorders in first degree relatives of children and adolescents with obsessive compulsive disorder, *J Am Acad Child Adolesc Psych* (1990) **29**: 407–12.

27 Pauls D, Alsobrook J, Goodman W et al, A family study of obsessive-compulsive disorder. *Am J Psychiatry* (1995) **152**:76–84.

28. Luxemberg J, Swedo S, Flament M et al, Neuroanatomical abnormalities in obsessive-compulsive disorder detected with quantitative X-ray computed tomography, *Am J Psychiatry* (1988) **145**:1089–93.

29 Rosenberg DR, Keshavan MS, Toward a neurodevelopmental model of obsessive-compulsive disorder, *Biol Psychiatry* (1998) **43**:623–40.

30 Cottraux J, Gérard D, Neuroimaging and neuroanatomical issues in obsessive-cognitive disorder. In: *Obsessive-compulsive Disorder: Theory, Research, and Treatment* Guilford Press: New York (1998): 154–80.

31 Swedo S, Shapiro M, Grady C et al, Cerebral glucose metabolism in childhood obsessive-compulsive disorder, *Arch Gen Psychiatry* (1989) **46**:518–23.

32. Swedo S, Pietrini P, Leonard H et al, Cerebral glucose metabolism in childhood obsessive-compulsive disorder: revisualization during pharmacotherapy, *Arch Gen Psychiatry* (1992) **49**:690–4.

33 Swedo SE, Rapoport JL, Cheslow DL et al, High prevalence of obsessive-compulsive symptoms in patients with Sydenham's chorea, *Am J Psychiatry* (1989) **146**:246–9.

34 Asbahr FR., Negrao AB, Gentil V et al, Obsessive-compulsive and related symptoms in children and adolescents with rheumatic fever with and without chorea: a prospective 6-month study, *Am J Psychiatry* (1998) **155**:1122–4.

35 Swedo S, Leonard HL, Garvey M et al, Pediatric autoimmune neuropsychiatric disorders associated with streptococcal infections (PANDAS): clinical description of the first 50 cases, *Am J Psychiatry* (1998) **155**:264–71.

36 Perlmutter SJ, Leitman SF, Garvey MA et al, Therapeutic plasma exchange and intravenous immunoglobulin for obsessive-compulsive disorder and tic disorders in childhood, *Lancet* (1999) **354**:1153–8.

37 Garvey MA, Perlmutter SJ, Allen AJ et al, A pilot study of penicillin prophylaxis for neuropsychiatric exacerbations triggered by streptococcal infections, *Biol Psychiatry* (1999) **45**:1564–71.

38 Flament MF, Rapoport JL, Berg CJ et al, Clomipramine treatment of childhood obsessive-compulsive disorder. A double-blind controlled study, *Arch Gen Psychiatry* (1985) **42**:977–83.

39 DeVeaugh-Geiss J, Moroz G, BieTderman J et al, Clomipramine hydrochloride in childhood and adolescent obsessive-compulsive disorder: a multicenter trial, *J Am Acad Child Adolesc Psych* (1992) **31**:45–9.

40 Leonard HL, Swedo SE, Rapoport JL et al, Treatment of obsessive-compulsive disorder with clomipramine and desipramine in children and adolescents, *Arch Gen Psychiatry* (1989) **46**:1088–92.

41 Flament MF, Rapoport JL, Murphy DL et al, Biochemical changes during clomipramine treatment of childhood obsessive compulsive disorder, *Arch Gen Psychiatry* (1987) **44**:219–25.

42 Riddle MA, Scahill L, King RA et al, Double-blind, crossover trial of fluoxetine and placebo in children and adolescents with obsessive-compulsive disorder, *J Am Acad Child Adolesc Psych* (1992) **31**:1062–9.

43 Apter A, Ratzoni G, King RA et al, Fluvoxamine open-label treatment of adolescent inpatients with obsessive-compulsive disorder or depression, *J Am Acad Child Adolesc Psych* (1994) **33**:342–8.

44. Thomsen PH, Child and adolescent obssesive-compulsive disorder treated with citalopram: findings from an open trial of 23 cases, *J Child Adolesc Psychopharmacol* (1997) **7**:157–66.

45 Rosenberg DR, Stewart CM, Fitzgerald KD et al, Paroxetine open-label treatment of pediatric outpatients with obsessive-compulsive disorder, *J Am Acad Child Adolesc Psych* (1999) **38**:1180–5.

46 March JS, Biederman J, Wolkow R et al, Sertraline in children and adolescents with obsessive-compulsive disorder: a multicenter randomized controlled trial, *JAMA* (1998) **280**:1752–6.

47 Leonard HL, Swedo SE, Lenane MC et al, A double-blind desipramine substitution during long-term clomipramine treatment in children and adolescents with obsessive-compulsive disorder, *Arch Gen Psychiatry* (1991) **48**:922–7.

48 March JS, Cognitive-behavioral psychotherapy for children and adolescents with OCD: a review and recommendations for treatment, *J Am Acad Child Adolesc Psych* (1995) **34**:7–18.

49 Bolton D, Collins S, Steinberg D, The treatment of obsessive-compulsive disorder in adolescence. A report of fifteen cases, *Br J Psychiatry* (1983) **142**:456–64.

50 March JS, Mulle K, Herbel B, Behavioral psychotherapy for children and adolescents with obsessive-compulsive disorder: an open trial of a new protocol-driven treatment package, *J Am Acad Child Adolesc Psych* (1994) **33**:333–41.

51 Franklin ME, Kozak MJ, Cashman L et al, Cognitive-behavioral treatment of pediatric obsessive compulsive disorder: an open clinical trial. *J Am Acad Child Adolesc Psych* (1998) **37**:412–19.

52 De Haan E, Hoogduin KA, Buitelaar JK, Keijsers G, Behavior therapy versus clomipramine for the treatment of obsessive-compulsive disorder in children and adolescents, *J Am Acad Child Adolesc Psych* (1998), **37**:1022–9.

53 Apter A, Bernhout E, Tyano S, Severe obsessive compulsive disorder in adolescence: a report of eight cases, *J Adolesc* (1984) **7**:349–58.

54 Target M, Fonagy P, Efficacy of psychoanalysis for children with emotional disorders, *J Am Acad Child Adolesc Psych* (1994) **33**:361–71.

55 Lenane M, Family therapy for children with obsessive-compulsive disorder. In: *Current Treatments of Obsessive-compulsive Disorder – Clinical Practice* Washington DC, Pato M, Zohar M, eds, American Psychiatric Association: 103–13.

56 Warren W, Some relationships between the psychiatry of children and adults, *J Ment Sci* (1960) **106**:815–26.

57 Leonard HL, Swedo SE, Lenane MC et al, A 2- to 7-year follow-up study of 54 obsessive-compulsive children and adolescents, *Arch Gen Psychiatry* (1993) **50**:429–39.

58 Bolton D, Luckie M, Steinberg D, Long-term course of obsessive-compulsive disorder treated in adolescence, *J Am Acad Child Adolesc Psych* (1995) **34**: 1441–50.

59 Thomsen PH, Mikkelsen HU, Obsessive-compulsive disorder in children and adolescents: predictors in childhood for long-term phenomenological course, *Acta Psychiatr Scand* (1995) **92**:255–9.

13
An integrated approach to the treatment of OCD

Dan J Stein, Naomi Fineberg and Soraya Seedat

Obsessive compulsive disorder (OCD) is, arguably, the psychiatric disorder that best exemplifies an integrated 'brain–mind' approach to the understanding of psychopathology. Previous chapters have covered aspects of the psychobiology of OCD; in particular, questions about the neuroanatomical, neurochemical and cognitive mechanisms mediating obsessional and compulsive symptoms have been explored. In this chapter we use this range of findings to provide a framework for an integrated approach to the treatment of OCD.

What is the core psychobiological deficit in OCD?

An integrated approach to the treatment of OCD would ideally rest on the basis of a clear understanding of the nature of the core psychobiological deficit underlying the disorder. Despite significant neurobiological advances in the field, defining a core psychobiological deficit in OCD remains an ambitious undertaking. As a first step towards this goal, we would tentatively suggest that the fundamental deficiency in OCD revolves around faults in the selection, maintenance and termination of 'procedural strategies', particularly (but not exclusively) those involving harm assessment.

Cortico–striatal–thalamic–cortical circuits and OCD

This characterization requires some unpacking. We can begin by recalling that the bulk of current evidence – neuropsychological, neuroimaging, neuroimmunological, and neurosurgical – emphasizes the role of cortico–striatal–thalamic–cortical (CSTC) dysfunction in OCD.[1,2] the immediate question, then, is what is the normal role of these circuits? The answer might be a clue to the nature of the core dysfunction in OCD.

It is widely believed that CSTC circuits play a role in organizing motor and cognitive procedural strategies.[3–5] Take, for example, the procedure for riding a bicycle. When we initially learn to ride, the effort requires a good deal of conscious concentration. However, over time, the brain–mind encodes a 'bicycling procedure' – this procedure is enacted non-consciously and automatically – under the direction of the striatum. Even when we lose our explicit memories of learning to ride a bicycle, our implicit knowledge of how to ride remains (this kind of dissociation has been documented, for example, in studies of dementia).

There is evidence suggesting that the neural mechanisms underlying procedural knowledge are disrupted in OCD. For example, when undertaking an implicit cognition task during functional brain imaging, normal controls demonstrated activation of CSTC circuits (especially striatum), but OCD patients showed a pathological activation of temporal regions instead.[6] Of course, OCD is not a dysfunction in bicycling; rather, OCD typically involves procedures that involve the assessment of harm. Thus, although OCD has been suggested to be a disorder of grooming (and some associated symptoms, such as tics, are primarily motoric), in patients with cleaning rituals there are invariably concerns about the harm of contamination.

The fact that the orbitofrontal cortex rather than the amygdala is predominantly activated in brain imaging studies of OCD suggests that the stimuli that generate anxiety for the OCD sufferer originate internally rather than externally. In contrast, in post-traumatic stress disorder (PTSD) a loud noise may stimulate thalamo–amygdaloid activation and produce an implicit, automatic fear response (startle reaction, etc.). It is postulated that in OCD, once a trigger – say a speck of dirt – has been noticed, an internal cognitive process, perhaps comprising disrupted or inefficient striatal processing, results in the exaggeration of its potential harmful consequences.

Core deficit vs compensatory dysfunctions

Although it is possible that increased orbitofrontal activation represents a primary lesion in OCD, there is increasing support for the idea that it is instead a compensatory response. In this view, orbitofrontal activation represents a compensatory reaction to dysfunction in subcortical structures, along the lines of a 'natural defence' against obsessional anxiety. Thus, increased activity in the orbitofrontal cortex may be an attempt to suppress striatally mediated harm exaggeration in OCD. It has been suggested that one of the roles of treatment may be to bolster this 'natural defence' mechanism.

The finding that OCD patients with low orbitofrontal activity prior to treatment are less likely to respond to medication is in line with this hypothesis.[7] It is as if there is not enough capacity in the system for adequate compensation to be achieved. Similarly, it is interesting that the behavioural exacerbation of OCD by sumatriptan, a specific agonist of the terminal autoreceptor (5-HT$_{1D}$) appears associated with decreased activity in areas of prefrontal cortex,[8] perhaps suggesting that the level of activity in the compensatory circuitry has been turned down by the drug.

Neurochemical theories and OCD

The neurochemical abnormalities found in OCD appear consistent with a hypothesis involving striatal dysfunction and abnormalities in procedures involving harm assessment, with orbitofrontal activation as a compensatory phenomenon. Both the striatum and the frontal cortex receive a rich innervation from serotonergic neurons, and a number of studies have begun to explore the interaction between neuroanatomical and neurochemical systems in OCD.[8,9]

It is notable that certain serotonergic systems appear underactive in OCD[10,11] as well as in impulsivity[11] (e.g. blunted prolactin response to the serotonergic agonist methyl-chlorophenylpiperazine (mCPP). The cognitive process whereby a speck of dirt triggers exaggerated fear of harm (by contamination) and sets off handwashing compulsions may well reflect striatal serotonergic hypofunction. Conversely, there is also evidence of hyperserotonergic function in OCD (e.g. enhanced growth hormone responses to L-tryptophan and D-fenfluramine,[12,13] symptom exacerbation after mCPP),[10,14] and this may represent prefrontal compensatory mechanisms at work.

This view of underlying deficit and secondary compensation in OCD provides a speculative way of tying together a range of neuroanatomical and neurochemical findings. But does it make sense in terms of our clinical understanding of the symptomatology and experience of suffering from OCD?

Psychodynamic theories and OCD

One of the most convincing descriptions of the phenomenology of OCD turns out to be that of Freud. Indeed, Freud's understanding of obsessional neurosis provides a cornerstone for psychodynamic theory, and is consistent with much modern thinking about the operation of an unconscious. For Freud, at the heart of obsessional neurosis are unconscious aggressive instincts.[15] Unacceptable urges, particularly hostile urges, are admitted into awareness because of incomplete repression, necessitating defensive responses in the form of compulsive rituals to reduce guilt and anxiety.

This formulation is redolent of the psychobiological characterization provided in the previous section. In OCD there may be a non-conscious, striatally mediated impulsive/disinhibited process. This results in frontally mediated compensatory attempts to switch this process off. A range of more recent data support a link between OCD and behavioural disinhibition. Epidemiological data indicate that OCD is frequently associated with a history of childhood impulsivity and aggression.[16] Furthermore, in clinical settings, individuals with OCD often demonstrate a degree of impulsive-aggression,[11] which, given their harm avoidance, is counterintuitively high.

More cognitive models: the role of doubt

So far we have concentrated on the central theme of harm assessment in OCD. Other authors, such as Tallis,[17] have drawn attention to the role of doubt in this disorder. According to Freud, doubt leads the patient to uncertainty about his protective measures, and to his continual repetition of them in order to banish that uncertainty. It is as though obsessional patients have lost the ability to register they have done something, or even to 'know if they know something'.[18]

It has been suggested that dysfunction of CSTC circuits may interfere with the normal verification of the successful completion of preventative or reparative behaviours, leading to compulsive repetition of the behaviours until appropriate information processing is accomplished.[19] Just how the compulsion eventually stops is not clear; perhaps the energy dissipates a little like that of a tuning fork.

An integrated approach to treatment

If the core psychobiological dysfunction in OCD revolves around striatally mediated problems in the selection, maintenance and termination of procedural strategies, how might we approach treatment?

First, serotonergic medication can be used to optimize striatal function, either by direct action at receptors in the striatum, or by augmenting orbitostriatal compensatory mechanisms as described above. Where striatal damage is more extensive, dopamine blockers may provide an additional mechanism for increased serotonergic neuronal activity, since dopaminergic neurons act to inhibit striatal serotonergic neurons.[20]

Second, cognitive-behavioural techniques can be used to regulate striatal function. For some reason, exposure to feared stimuli, like pharmacotherapy, ultimately results in optimization of the CSTC circuits. Baxter's elegant work showing comparable effects of a selective serotonin reuptake inhibitor and behavioural therapy on the functional neuroanatomy of OCD, remains a key finding propelling forward the idea of an integrated brain–mind approach to OCD.[21]

Third, there may be a range of preventative interventions that can be applied, early in life, to protect the striatum. The basal ganglia are particularly vulnerable to neonatal hypoxaemia, and preventing this is therefore important. The finding that childhood emotional deprivation is associated with neuroanatomical abnormalities in the striatum provides an even more challenging area for therapeutic intervention.[22]

Finally, autoimmune processes in the aftermath of streptococcal infection may also result in striatal damage.[23] It will be interesting to see whether prophylactic measures including aggressive early diagnosis and intervention with antibiotics are ultimately able to have a positive impact on the occurrence and course of Paediatric Autoimmune Neuropsychiatric Disorders Associated with *Streptococcus* (PANDAS).[24]

Are integrated treatments more effective in OCD?

We know that serotonin reuptake inhibitors (SRIs) and behaviour therapy are individually effective in OCD, and it would therefore seem likely that the combination of both treatments would provide even better efficacy. In fact, there have been few studies looking at this area, and the evidence to date remains incomplete.[25] Meta-analyses, such as that by Picinelli et al,[26] have not succeeded in addressing the question of relative efficacy of interventions, partly because this kind of statistical approach cannot adequately correct for the changes that have occurred between individual trials over the years, such as rising placebo response rates during the 1990s and the greater numbers of treatment-resistant and atypical patients entering later medication trials. Head-to-head comparisons of the effects of combination treatment versus drug or behavioural monotherapy are preferable, and it is regrettable that so few properly controlled studies have been performed.

Early influential studies by Marks and colleagues were the first to address the question of how best to sequence and combine pharmacotherapy and psychotherapy in OCD.[27,28] Their first study suggested that the addition of clomipramine to behaviour therapy enhanced compliance and produced a more favourable outcome.[27] These results were echoed in a second study, where the addition of clomipramine to exposure therapy produced a greater level of improvement.[28] Unfortunately these studies are limited by a number of methodological problems, including the use of small sample sizes.

A study by Kozac, Liebowitz and Foa (personal communication) investigating the clinical effectiveness of cognitive-behavioural psychotherapy, pharmacotherapy and combination therapy in a large group of patients was initiated, but did not develop into a full trial. However, two small studies by Cottraux et al and Hohagen et al have been reported in full.[29,30] Both studies compared fluvoxamine plus behaviour therapy with placebo plus behaviour therapy, and, in spite of small numbers, demonstrated superior efficacy for the combination over exposure monotherapy for up to 6 months. There was no drug monotherapy arm in one of the studies.[30] The study by Cottraux et al was unable to show a significant advantage for combined drug and exposure compared with fluvoxamine, even though the drug was given in combination with antiexposure (which should have had an adverse effect), but the study was probably under-powered (n = 40), and the authors themselves advocated further, larger studies.[29]

All in all, it may be concluded that there is benefit to be gained by adding drug treatment to exposure therapy, but it is rather less clear whether combining drug treatment with exposure is any more effective than drug treatment given alone. Optimistic claims from uncontrolled case series that cognitive-behaviour therapy prevents relapse if medica-tion is prematurely discontinued (e.g. March et al),[31] although intuitively persuasive, need to be explored further under properly controlled conditions.

An integrated approach in practice

So far this chapter has been rather theoretical. How does an integrated approach work in practice?

The first step of treatment is a comprehensive psychiatric and medical history and examination. Particular symptoms in OCD (such as tics) and comorbid disorders (such as depression) may well influence the choice of intervention. Evaluation of OCD symptoms with a scale such as the Yale–Brown Obsessive Compulsive Scale (see Appendix 1, p. 183) is useful in determining treatment targets. During these initial interactions with the patient, conveying an empathic appreciation of the experience of OCD is crucial for strengthening the clinician–patient relationship, and this kind of effect may even have contributed to the efficacy of placebo in recent clinical trials. Patients are often relieved to realize from the direc-tion of the clinician's questions that other patients also suffer from intensely embarrassing symptoms (such as intrusive sexual obsessions).

Once the patient has been appropriately evaluated and diagnosed it is important to begin a process of psychoeducation. In many ways, this is the first step of cognitive-behavioural treatment. It is useful to begin by asking patients for their 'explanatory model' of OCD – what are their ideas about the cause of their symptoms?[32] Often people misconstrue symptoms as reflecting unconscious guilt, or as pointing towards a hid-den personality fault. The shame that is associated with the experience of OCD (e.g. feeling incompetent for being unable to control an ego-dystonic compulsion) is presumably one of the reasons for the long lag time between first experiencing OCD symptoms and seeking treatment.[33] The clinician can present an alternative view of OCD as a striatal 'false alarm' (as outlined in different words above) and then negotiate with the patient to try to achieve a shared understanding and treatment plan.

The use of psychoeducation raises the question of consumer advocacy; this would seem increasingly relevant to an integrated approach to the treatment of OCD. Modern media allow for rapid communication of ideas, and for bringing together clinicians and consumers electronically. Stigmatization of mental illness can be addressed by providing appropriate information, referral to support groups, etc. Virtual support groups can also be immensely useful for people with OCD.[34] Given the early onset of OCD symptoms, there would seem to be a need to target information about OCD and other psychiatric disorders to youngsters and to professionals such as teachers who are most often in contact with this population.

Once treatment itself begins, either medication or cognitive-behavioural therapy can be chosen, depending on a range of factors including symptom severity, comorbid illness (e.g. depression), and patient choice. (We use the term 'cognitive-behavioural therapy' as cognitive interventions may also have a role in the treatment of OCD, although the majority of evidence for the efficacy of psychotherapy in OCD has focused on the value of exposure per se). Despite the relatively limited database discussed earlier, most clinicians conservatively advocate combined pharmacotherapy and psychotherapy, if available, for the majority of OCD patients. If medication is to be discontinued, it would seem wise to do this gradually over a period of months, and to stress again the principles of exposure therapy during this time.

Drug treatment is generally available and can be monitored by a primary care practitioner, except where unusually high doses of medication or augmentation strategies are employed. Cognitive-behavioural therapy for OCD is generally less accessible and usually requires referral to a specialist centre, where there are often long waiting lists for treatment. However, the psychotherapy component of exposure therapy is not difficult to learn, and can be taught to a range of mental-health professionals. Indeed, there seems to be a demand from community psychiatric nurses to learn these skills.

Next, it is useful to incorporate the family and significant others into the treatment plan. It is important, for example, to assess the adverse effects of the patient's symptoms on family function.[35] Furthermore, behavioural techniques may not be effective when the family works (sometimes in good faith) to prevent exposure. For example, when a patient with contamination concerns has an equally fastidious spouse, there is often mutual reinforcement to exclude exposure, and the couple must therefore be treated together.

In refractory patients, partial or full hospitalization may be a useful option for ensuring that both optimal pharmacotherapy and psychotherapy are given.[36] Referral to a specialist unit for OCD where both forms of treatment (as well as expertise in neurosurgery) are available should be considered in patients who have failed initial pharmacotherapy, psychotherapy, or combined treatments. Fortunately, however, the majority of people with OCD can be treated on an outpatient basis and will respond to simple combinations of psychoeducation, an SRI and exposure therapy.

Conclusion

Although much remains to be understood about the neurobiology of OCD, there is a convergence on certain hypotheses, and striatal dysfunction seems particularly important. Remarkably, both psychotherapy and pharmacotherapy result in normalization of striatal function. Taken together, this means that OCD provides an extraordinarily powerful model of a contemporary approach to the brain–mind, to psychopathology, and to treatment. In the clinical setting it is useful to be able to educate the patient that the 'false alarm' in their brain–mind can be reset through a combination of pharmacotherapy and exposure. For researchers, determining the precise mechanisms through which these interventions operate remains an exciting challenge.

References

1 Rauch SL, Baxter LR, Neuroimaging in obsessive-compulsive disorder and related disorders. In: Jenicke MA, Baer L, Minichiello WE (eds) *Obsessive-Compulsive Disorders: Practice Management*, (3rd edn) (Mosby: St Louis, 1998).

2 Stein DJ, Goodman WK, Rauch SL, The cognitive-affective neuroscience of obsessive-compulsive disorder, *Current Psychiatric Rev* (2000) **2**:341–6.

3 Cummings JL, Frontal-subcortical circuits and human behavior. *Arch Neurol* (1993) **50**:873–80.

4 Robbins TW, Brown VJ, The role of the striatum in the mental chronometry of action: a theoretical review, *Rev Neurosci* (1990) **2**:181–213.

5 Saint-Cyr JA, Taylor AE, Nicholson K, Behavior and the basal ganglia. In: WJ Weiner, AE Lang (eds) *Behavioral Neurology of Movement Disorders* (Raven Press: New York, 1995).

6 Rauch SL, Savage CR, Alpert NM et al, Probing striatal function in obsessive compulsive disorder: a PET study of implicit sequence learning, *J Neuropsychiatry* (1997) **9**:568–73.

7 Swedo SE, Pietrini P, Leonard HL et al, Cerebral glucose metabolism in childhood-onset obsessive-compulsive disorder: revisualization during pharmacotherapy, *Arch Gen Psychiatry* (1992) **49**:690–4.

8 Stein DJ, van Heerden B, Wessels CJ et al, Single photon emission tomography of the brain with Tc-99m HMPAO during sumatriptan challenge in obsessive-compulsive disorder: investigating the functional role of the serotonin auto-receptor, *Prog Neuropsychopharmacol Biol Psychiatry* (1999) **23**:1079–99.

9 Hollander E, Prohovnik I, Stein DJ, Obsessions and cerebral blood flow during pharmacological challenge with m-CPP, *J Neuropsychiatr Clin Neurosci* (1995) **7**:485–90.

10 Zohar J, Mueller EA, Insel TR et al, Serotonergic responsivity in obsessive-compulsive disorder: comparison of patients and healthy controls, *Arch Gen Psychiatry* (1987) **44**:946–51.

11 Stein DJ, Hollander E, Impulsive aggression and obsessive-compulsive disorder, *Psychiatr Ann* (1993) **23**:389–95.

12 Fineberg NA, Montgomery SA, Cowen PJ, Neuroendocrine responses to intravenous L-tryptophan in obsessive compulsive disorder, *J Affect Disord* (1994) **32**:97–104.

13 Fineberg NA, Roberts A, Montgomery SA, Cowan PJ, Brain 5-HT function in obsessive compulsive disorder. Prolactin responses to d-fenfluramine, *Br J Psychiatry* (1997) **171**:280–2.

14 Hollander E, DeCaria C, Nitescu A et al, Serotonergic function in obsessive compulsive disorder: behavioral and neuroendocrine responses to oral m-CPP and fenfluramine in patients and healthy volunteers, *Arch Gen Psychiatry* (1992) **49**:21–8.

15 Freud S, Inhibitions, symptoms and anxiety. (1926) *Standard Edition of the Complete Psychological Works of Sigmund Freud*, vol. 20 (Hogarth Press: London) 111–31.

16 Hollander E, Stein DJ, Broatch J, Himelein C, Rowland C, A pharmacoeconomic and quality of life study of obsessive-compulsive disorder, *CNS Spectr* (1997) **2**: 16–25.

17 Tallis F, *Obsessive Compulsive Disorder: A Cognitive and Neuropsychological Perspective* (John Wiley: Chichester, 1995).

18 Rapoport JL, *The Boy Who Couldn't Stop Washing: The Experience and Treatment of Obsessive Compulsive Disorder* (Dutton: New York, 1989).

19 Stein DJ, Hollander E, Cognitive science and obsessive-compulsive disorder. In: Stein DJ, Young JE (eds) *Cognitive Science and Clinical Disorders* (Academic Press: San Diego, 1992).

20 McDougle CJ, Goodman WK, Leckman JF et al, Haloperidol addition in fluvoxamine-refractory obsessive-compulsive disorder: a double-blind placebo-controlled study in patients with and without tics, *Arch Gen Psychiatry* (1994) **51**:302–8.

21 Baxter LR, Schwartz JM, Bergman KS et al, Caudate glucose metabolic rate changes with both drug and behavior therapy for OCD, *Arch Gen Psychiatry* (1992) **49**:681–9.

22 Martin LJ, Spicer DM, Lewis MH, Gluck JP, Cork LC, Social deprivation of infant monkeys alters the chemoarchitecture of the brain: I. Subcortical regions, *J Neurosci* (1991) **11**:3344–58.

23 Swedo SE, Leonard HL, Garvey M et al, Pediatric autoimmune neuropsychiatric disorders associated with streptococcal infections: clinical description of the first 50 cases, *Am J Psychiatry* (1998) **155**:264–71.

24 Garvey MA, Perlmutter SA, Allen AJ et al, A pilot study of penicillin prophylaxis for neuropsychiatric exacerbations triggered by streptococcal infections, *Biol Psychiatry* (1999) **45**:1564–71.

25 Fineberg N, Roberts A, Drummond L, Should we combine drug and exposure treatments in OCD? World Psychiatric Association: The Synthesis Between Psychopharmacology and Psychotherapy,

Jerusalem, Israel, 16–21 November 1997.

26   Picinelli M, Pini S, Bellatuono C et al, Efficacy of drug treatment in obsessive compulsive disorder, A meta-analytic review, *Br J Psychiatry* (1995) **166**:424–43.

27   Marks IM, Stern RS, Mawson D et al, Clomipramine and exposure for obsessive compulsive rituals. I, *Br J Psychiatry* (1980) **136**: 1–25.

28   Marks IM, Lelliott P, Basoglu M et al, Clomipramine, self exposure and therapist aided exposure for obsessive compulsive rituals, *Br J Psychiatry* (1988) **152**:522–34.

29   Cottraux J, Mollard E, Bouvard M et al, A controlled study of fluvoxamine and exposure in obsessive compulsive disorder, *Int Clin Psychopharmacol* (1990) **5**:17–30.

30   Hohagen F, Winkelmann G, Rasche-Rauchle H et al, Combination of behaviour therapy with fluvoxamine in comparison with behaviour therapy and placebo: results of a multicentre study, *Br J Psychiatry* (1998) **173**(suppl. 35): 71–8.

31   March JS, Mulle K, Herbel B. Behavioral psychotherapy for children and adolescents with obsessive compulsive disorder: an open trial of a new protocol driven treatment package, *J Am Acad Child Adolesc Psych* (1994) **33**:333–41.

32   Stein DJ, Rapoport JL, Cross-cultural studies and obsessive-compulsive disorder, *CNS Spectr* (1996) **1**:42–6.

33   Hollander E, Greenwald S, Neville D et al, Uncomplicated and comorbid obsessive-compulsive disorder in an epidemiological sample, *Depress Anxiety* (1996–7) **4**:111–19.

34   Stein DJ, Psychiatry on the internet: survey of an OCD mailing list, *Psychiatr Bull* (1996) **20**:1–4.

35   Calvocoressi L, Lewis B, Harris M et al, Family accommodation in obsessive-compulsive disorder, *Am J Psychiatry* (1995) **152**: 441–3.

36   Bystritsky A, Munford PR, Rosen RM et al, A preliminary study of partial hospital management of severe obsessive-compulsive disorder, *Psychiatr Serv* (1996) **47**:170–4.

14
Patients' perspectives on OCD

Frederick Toates

Abandoning modesty for a moment, I can claim to have a particular expertise on the subject of obsessive compulsive disorder (OCD), being both psychologist and sufferer. As a psychologist studying motivation, emotion and the control of behaviour, a probably fruitful, though not entirely welcome, cooperation is possible between two fundamental aspects of myself.

In 1973, somewhat in the fashion of a Woody Allen movie, I was overcome by intrusive, fearful and depressing obsessional thoughts about death and thereby the futility of a finite life. Although the appearance of these thoughts was sudden and dramatic, they came against a background of life-long chronic worry. On the one level, I could justify partly the contents of the intrusive thoughts in terms of rationality; they did not seem to be totally absurd. Indeed, the fact that Woody Allen can so effectively tap urban everyman's (and woman's) existential fears is indicative of this. However, what was clearly absurd and maladaptive was the frequency and intensity with which the intrusions came into conscious awareness.

In the following 27 years, having tried virtually every treatment, conventional and unconventional, I feel that I am in a good position to give some insights. First, I will present some personal reflections and review the insight that I gained from reactions to my autobiographical book. Then I will briefly wear the hat of an experimental psychologist to try to relate this to a scientific understanding.

Personal insight

Short of a miracle drug, a kind of chemical leucotomy, I accept that I shall probably never be completely cured. However, I can cope with it. I feel that there is a threshold, below which there exists a frequency and intensity of intrusion that is tolerable. One can cope in the sense that life has a net positive feel to it. When the frequency or intensity increases beyond a certain level, life takes a quantum leap in a negative direction.

On first seeking help I felt somewhat foolish discussing the problem with my doctor. It was not that he gave me any reason to feel odd, quite the contrary. I just wished that there were some recognized neural abnormality ('hardware') to which I could relate, rather than what appeared to be a 'software' programming fault. My hunch is that the advent of selective serotonin reuptake inhibitors (SSRIs) has given a number of people comfort in this direction.

Reactions to the book

After having published an autobiographical book about my experience with the disorder,[1] I was invited to appear on a number of television and radio programmes, some being interactive with 'phone-in' listeners. I also addressed self-help sufferers' groups. I was overwhelmed by the expressions of solidarity, concern and sympathy from fellow-sufferers. Some people let me know that they were praying for me.

To a number of people the book was 'open season' to speculate wildly about the causes of the problem – see, for example, the review by Kwee.[2] I even read that, unknown to me, I had been the victim of Satanic ritual abuse – and that appeared in an article originating in a British university! From colleagues came the message – 'We would never have known.' I even heard the occasional 'What is all the fuss about? Believe me – there is nothing wrong with you, you work and function normally – look at your work output.' My strong feeling is that, in spite of the demise of behaviourism as an explanatory tool in psychology, in reality people tend to judge others almost entirely by their outward behaviour. If behaviour looks right then the assumption is that there can be little wrong.

I was surprised at the number of people – considered by me to be 'healthily normal' – who came up to me for a quiet chat along the following lines: 'I have never told anyone about this before, but some years ago I found that I couldn't stop checking the door. But it went away after a month.' Somewhat disconcerting for me was the very occasional person (including one police officer) who reported the first appearance of (mercifully only transient) bouts of intrusive rumination triggered by reading about a particular theme in my book!

One lady summed up the essence of many comments: 'There is something particularly fascinating about being granted an insight into someone else's inner, mental life.' Virtually everyone congratulated me on the quality of courage in going public, which perhaps says something about the mind-set of people regarding acceptance of psychiatric disturbance.

I felt a sense of great responsibility and yet frustration in dealing with the people who wrote to me. I wished that I could have suggested a magic cure. Perhaps the clearest message to come from the sufferers was a feeling of isolation and oddness. Some had, up to then, felt sure that they alone had the condition. One man wrote:

> I felt like an alien. It was very difficult to believe that there were other people out there who were experiencing the same problems as I was and the great depressing rarely-receding pain. Now I feel like part of a club. Albeit a very odd club.

Some revealed just how well they had managed to camouflage their OCD. Very many asked me, in pleading terms, if there was any light at the end of the tunnel. Some were relieved to know that they were not psychotic. From a self-help group in Hampshire, I received the comment:

> Our group now refer to you as 'Fred' as I hope you don't mind us calling you and wish to congratulate you on your most interesting and comforting dialogue. We, as a group, know that we are not alone and are definitely not 'mad'.

The biggest comfort from the book was that readers felt less odd that someone had gone public. A number said that they felt they were misunderstood souls struggling against prejudice, and they hoped that an increase of information in the broader domain would help the general public gain greater understanding of the condition and become more accepting of it. It was highly significant to them that here was a personal angle, not simply that of an expert. Some appeared alienated from the world and were desperate for an intimate rapport. Others were comforted by common features such as a shared star-sign, hobby or county of birth. One lady even sent me a highlighted copy of my book, pointing out the sections and words most relevant to her. One man, an engine driver, drove down from Manchester and arrived at the university reception office, burst into tears and refused to go until he had talked to me. On more than one occasion I was told that the book had saved a life from suicide.

A number reported that, at last, they had found a recognized condition from which they suffer. It has a name and they are legitimate sufferers. A few people said that they felt more confident in describing the condition – something along the lines of 'I should have been able to tell all that to my doctor, but lacked the confidence and framework.' I seemed to form a frame of reference for them: 'Look – he is a successful academic and so I can't be so strange after all.' They would tell me, 'I found the book by accident and then I realized that's me exactly.' Some went to their doctors clutching my book as support for requesting an SSRI.

I also glimpsed the creative talent out there amongst sufferers and their families in terms of such things as attempts to provide augmented feedback about things checked. One family had devised a series of sticky labels to be attached each evening to doors and windows. These would then be peeled off by the checker and attached to a numbered board to be presented, on completion, to the partner. Similarly, the method of augmenting feedback in labelling checks that I employed on myself has been investigated as a therapeutic tool and there are suggestions that it is useful for some people.[3,4]

A number reported their despair at trying one thing after another with no tangible results. A significant number reported great difficulty getting the right professional help – feeling themselves to be treated as oddballs and misunderstood. Several said that they had not talked to anyone about their condition, believing that they were alone or that no help could be obtained. Some people asked for reassurance, putting me almost in the role of guru: 'Well, you must be able to convince me that I am not evil.' A number sent their life histories in page after page of detailed account. Perhaps not surprisingly, obsessionals are nothing if not good diarists and documenters!

My clear impression was that, in many cases, OCD sprang from a context of stress and conflict, for example existential crises on the meaning of life, abuse, drug addiction and unemployment.

In terms of access to treatment, regional variations became evident both in the UK and, based on a couple of letters, in France. Professionals often did not know what to do. The proximity to a good centre with an understanding therapist seemed out of reach to many.

Amongst therapists the book was generally well received. However, one reviewer (Kwee) suggested that it might give a misleading impression that 'quick fixes' such as behaviour therapy and chemical cures are viable.[2] He suggested that the OC personality needs untangling. Another reviewer said that she would be reluctant to recommend the book to her patients on the grounds that it might increase their despair: if a psychologist can't get cured, what hope is there for them?

So can such personal experience mesh with scientific insight?

Links with a scientific approach

A number of authors have suggested that behaviour is the product of parallel processes of control.[5,6] Crudely dichotomized, these can be characterized by (a) relatively fast, 'on-line', direct, inflexible, stimulus-response (S–R) links, and (b) slower, 'off-line', indirect, flexible, cognitive processes.[7,8] The resultant behaviour represents the resolution of these two influences, which can cooperate or, at times, be in conflict. With development, learning or brain damage, the relative weight of these factors can change. Thought itself also appears to be the product of a similar set of parallel processes.[9,10] Could such a model be useful for understanding OCD?

My own phenomenological experience would suggest that it can. At times, thoughts appear to be triggered directly by particular appropriate stimuli, such as seeing an assassination attempt on television. Conversely, sometimes they appear to be cued by a suggestion of resolution: now things look good, that particular problem is solved. It feels as if there is a queue for processing space, and resolution of a temporary problem permits the obsessional thought to take over.

At other times, negative thoughts appear to pop into consciousness without external trigger cues. Rather, they seem to be a result of work going on at an unconscious level. It seems as if they are tagged at this level 'for further attention' or 'pending' and cannot be assimilated into the vast array of memories held in a relatively inaccessible form. Some theories of consciousness see a limited and expensive workspace as being the arena into which material is brought which has failed to be resolved at a lower level.[11] This is how it feels to me.

There is a growing appreciation of the role of feedback from the body in determining central mood and emotion.[12-14] My own feeling is that such general factors might bias cognition in a negative direction. Hence, stress quite unrelated to the disorder might exacerbate it. Diet could even do this if it induces gastrointestinal discomfort.

Conclusion

I hope that phenomonological observation of the sufferer on his or her own conscious mind and behaviour can be assimilated into more conventional approaches. It would seem an obvious way forward. In his foreword to my book, Hans Eysenck expressed the wish that other psychologists would come forward with details of their troubles. One such is Chadwick, who has written on the topic of paranoia.[15]

Acknowledgement

I am grateful to Dr Richard Stevens of the Open University for his comments.

References

1 Toates F, *Obsessional Thoughts and Behaviour* (Thorsons: Wellingborough, 1990). Reprinted as *Obsessive-Compulsive Disorder* (Thorsons: London, 1992).

2 Kwee M, Book review, *Behav Res Ther* (1991) **29**:371–3.

3 Tallis F, Doubt reduction using distinctive stimuli as a treatment for compulsive checking: an exploratory investigation, *Clin Psychol Psychother* (1993) **1**: 45–52.

4 Watts FN, An information-processing approach to compulsive checking. *Clin Psychol Psychother* (1995) **2**:69–77.

5 Hirsh R, The hippocampus and

contextual retrieval of information from memory: a theory, *Behav Biol* (1974) **12**:421–44.

6 Le Doux J, *The Emotional Brain* (Weidenfeld & Nicolson: London, 1998).

7 Toates F, The interaction of cognitive and stimulus-response processes in the control of behaviour. *Neurosci Biobehav Rev* (1998) **22**:59–83.

8 Toates F, *Biological Psychology: An Integrative Approach* (Prentice-Hall: Harlow, 2001).

9 Epstein S, Integration of the cognitive and the psychodynamic unconscious, *Am Psychol* (1994) **49**:709–24.

10 Sloman SA, The empirical case for two systems of reasoning, *Psychol Bull* (1996) **119**:3–22.

11 Baars BJ, *In the Theater of Consciousness*, (Oxford University Press: New York, 1997).

12 Damasio AR, *Descartes' Error* (Papermac: London, 1996).

13 Rosenbaum JF, Heninger G, Vagus nerve stimulation for treatment-resistant depression, *Biol Psychiatry* (2000) **47**:273–5.

14 Rush AJ, George MS, Sackeim HA et al, Vagus nerve stimulation (VNS) for treatment-resistant depressions: a multicenter study, *Biol Psychiatry* (2000) **47**:276–86.

15 Chadwick P, The stepladder to the impossible: a first hand phenomenological account of a schizoaffective psychotic crisis, *J Ment Health* (1993) **2**:239–50.

Appendix 1: Major rating scales

Yale–Brown Obsessive Compulsive Scale (YBOCS)*†

General instructions

This rating scale is designed to rate the severity and type of symptoms in patients with obsessive-compulsive disorder (OCD). In general, the items depend on the patient's report; however, the final rating is based on the clinical judgment of the interviewer. Rate the characteristics of each item during the prior week up until and including the time of the interview. Scores should reflect the average (mean) occurrence of each item for the entire week.

This rating scale is intended for use as a semistructured interview. The interviewer should assess the items in the listed order and use the questions provided. However, the interviewer is free to ask additional questions for purposes of clarification. If the patient volunteers information at any time during the interview, that information will be considered. Ratings should be based primarily on reports and observations gained during the interview. If you judge that the information being provided is grossly inaccurate, then the reliability of the patient is in doubt and should be noted accordingly at the end of the interview (item 19).

Additional information supplied by others (e.g., spouse or parent) may be included in a determination of the ratings only if it is judged that (1) such information is essential to adequately assessing symptom severity *and* (2) consistent week-to-week reporting can be ensured by having the same informant(s) present for each rating session.

Before proceeding with the questions, define 'obsessions' and 'compulsions' for the patient as follows:

Obsessions are unwelcome and distressing ideas, thoughts, images or impulses that repeatedly enter your mind. They may seem to occur against your will. They may be repugnant to you, you may recognize them as senseless, and they may not fit your personality.

Compulsions, on the other hand, are behaviors or acts that you feel driven to perform, although you may recognize them as senseless or

*Developed by Wayne K Goodman, MD. *Steven A Rasmussen, MD, Lawrence H Price, MD, Carolyn Mazure, PhD, George R Heninger, MD, Dennis S Charney, MD, Department of Psychiatry, Yale University School of Medicine, and *Department of Psychiatry, Brown University School of Medicine. Used by permission.
†First Edition 7/86; revised 9/89.
Copyright Wayne K Goodman, MD, 1989

excessive. At times, you may try to resist doing them but this may prove difficult. You may experience anxiety that does not diminish until the behavior is completed.

Let me give you some examples of obsessions and compulsions.

An example of an obsession is the recurrent thought or impulse to do serious physical harm to your children even though you never would.

An example of a compulsion is the need to repeatedly check appliances, water faucets, and the lock on the front door before you can leave the house. While most compulsions are observable behaviors, some are unobservable mental acts, such as silent checking or having to recite nonsense phrases to yourself each time you have a bad thought.

Do you have any questions about what these words mean?

[If not, proceed.]

On repeated testing it is not always necessary to reread these definitions and examples as long as it can be established that the patient understands them. It may be sufficient to remind the patient that obsessions are the thoughts or concerns and compulsions are the things you feel driven to do, including covert mental acts.

Have the patient enumerate current obsessions and compulsions in order to generate a list of target symptoms. Use the YBOCS Symptom Checklist as an aid for identifying current symptoms. It is also useful to identify and be aware of past symptoms since they may reappear during subsequent ratings. Once the current types of obsessions and compulsions are identified, organize and list them on the Target Symptoms form according to clinically convenient distinctions (e.g., divide target compulsions into checking and washing). Describe salient features of the symptoms so that they can be more easily tracked (e.g., in addition to listing checking, specify what the patient checks for). Be sure to indicate which are the most prominent symptoms (i.e., those that will be the major focus of assessment). Note, however, that the final score for each item should reflect a composite rating of all of the patient's obsessions or compulsions.

The rater must ascertain whether reported behaviors are bona fide symptoms of OCD and not symptoms of another disorder, such as simple phobia or a paraphilia. The differential diagnosis between certain complex motor tics and certain compulsions (e.g., involving touching) may be difficult or impossible. In such cases, it is particularly important to provide explicit descriptions of the target symptoms and to be consistent in subsequent ratings. Separate assessment of tic severity with a tic rating instrument may be necessary in such cases. Some of the items listed on the YBOCS Symptom Checklist, such as trichotillomania, are currently classified in DSM-III-R as symptoms of an impulse control disorder. It should be noted that the suitability of the YBOCS for use in disorders other than DSM-III-R–defined OCD has yet to be established. However, when using the YBOCS to rate severity of symptoms not strictly classified under OCD (e.g., trichotillomania) in a patient who otherwise meets criteria for OCD, it has been our practice to administer the YBOCS twice; once for conventional obsessive-compulsive symptoms and a second time for putative OCD-related phenomena. In this fashion separate YBOCS scores are generated for severity of OCD and severity of other symptoms in which the relationship to OCD is still unsettled.

On repeated testing, review and, if necessary, revise target obsessions prior to rating item 1. Do likewise for compulsions prior to rating item 6.

All 19 items are rated, but only items 1–10 (excluding items 1b and 6b) are used to determine the total score. The total YBOCS score is the sum of items 1–10 (excluding 1b and 6b), whereas the obsession and compulsion subtotals are the sums of items 1–5 (excluding 1b) and 6–10 (excluding 6b), respectively.

Because at the time of this writing (9/89) there are limited data regarding the psychometric properties of items 1b, 6b, and 11–16, these items should be considered investigational. Until adequate studies of the reliability, validity, and sensitivity to change of these items are conducted, we must caution against placing much weight on results derived from these item scores. These important caveats aside, we believe that items 1b (obsession-free interval), 6b (compulsion-free interval), and 12 (avoidance) may provide information that has bearing on the severity of obsessive-compulsive symptoms. Item 11 (insight) may also furnish useful clinical information. We are least secure about the usefulness of items 13–16.

Items 17 (global severity) and 18 (global improvement) have been adapted from the Clinical Global Impression Scale to provide measures of overall functional impairment associated with, but not restricted to, the presence of obsessive-compulsive symptoms. Disability produced by secondary depressive symptoms would also be considered when rating these items. Item 19, which estimates the reliability of the information reported by the patient, may assist in the interpretation of scores on other YBOCS items in some cases of OCD.

See over for checklist.

YBOCS symptom checklist (9/89)

Name _____   Date _____

Check all that apply, but clearly mark the principal symptoms with a 'P.'
(Rater must ascertain whether reported behaviors are bona fide symptoms of
OCD, and not symptoms of another disorder such as simple phobia or
hypochondrias. Items marked '*' may or may not be OCD phenomena.)

Current	Past	
		Aggressive Obsessions
____	____	Fear might harm self
____	____	Fear might harm others
____	____	Violent or horrific images
____	____	Fear of blurting out obscenities or insults
____	____	Fear of doing something else embarrassing*
____	____	Fear will act on unwanted impulses (e.g., to stab friend)
____	____	Fear will steal things
____	____	Fear will harm others because not careful enough (e.g., hit/run MVA*)
____	____	Fear will be responsible for something else terrible happening (e.g., fire, burglary)
____	____	Other _____
		Contamination Obsessions
____	____	Concerns or disgust with bodily waste or secretions (e.g., urine, feces, saliva)
____	____	Concern with dirt or germs
____	____	Excessive concern with environment contaminants (e.g., asbestos, radiation, toxic waste)
____	____	Excessive concern with household items (e.g., cleaners, solvents)
____	____	Excessive concern with animals (e.g., insects)
____	____	Bothered by sticky substances or residues
____	____	Concerned will get ill because of contaminant
____	____	Concerned will get others ill by spreading contaminant (aggressive)
____	____	No concern with consequences of contamination other than how it might feel
____	____	Other _____
		Sexual Obsessions
____	____	Forbidden or perverse sexual thoughts, images, or impulses
____	____	Content involves children or incest
____	____	Content involves homosexuality*
____	____	Sexual behavior toward others (aggressive)*
____	____	Other _____
		Hoarding/Saving Obsessions
		[distinguish from hobbies and concern with objects of monetary or sentimental value]
____	____	

*MVA = motor vehicle accident

Religious Obsessions (scrupulosity)
____   ____   Concerned with sacrilege and blasphemy
____   ____   Excess concern with right/wrong, morality
____   ____   Other _____

Obsession with Need for Symmetry or Exactness
____   ____   Accompanied by magical thinking (e.g., concerned that mother
              will have accident unless things are in the right place)
____   ____   Not accompanied by magical thinking

Miscellaneous Obsessions
____   ____   Need to know or remember
____   ____   Fear of saying certain things
____   ____   Fear of not saying just the right thing
____   ____   Fear of losing things
____   ____   Intrusive (nonviolent) images
____   ____   Intrusive nonsense sounds, words, or music
____   ____   Bothered by certain sounds/noises*
____   ____   Lucky/unlucky numbers
____   ____   Colors with special significance
____   ____   Superstitious fears
____   ____   Others _____

Somatic Obsessions
____   ____   Concern with illness or disease*
____   ____   Excessive concern with body part or aspect of appearance
              (e.g., dysmorphophobia)*
____   ____   Other _____

Cleaning/Washing Compulsions
____   ____   Excessive or ritualized handwashing
____   ____   Excessive or ritualized showering, bathing, toothbrushing,
              grooming, or toilet routine
____   ____   Involves cleaning of household items or other inanimate objects
____   ____   Other measures to prevent or remove contact with
              contaminants
____   ____   Other _____

Checking Compulsions
____   ____   Checking locks, stove, appliances, etc.
____   ____   Checking that did not/will not harm others
____   ____   Checking that did not/will not harm self
____   ____   Checking that nothing terrible did/will happen
____   ____   Checking that did not make mistake
____   ____   Checking tied to somatic obsessions
____   ____   Other _____

Repeating Rituals
____   ____   Rereading or rewriting
____   ____   Need to repeat routine activities (e.g., in/out door, up/down
              from chair)
____   ____   Other _____

Counting Compulsions

____   ____   _____

Ordering/Arranging Compulsions

____   ____   _____

Hoarding/Collecting Compulsions
[distinguish from hobbies and concern with objects of monetary or sentimental value (e.g., carefully reads junk mail, piles up old newspapers, sorts through garbage, collects useless objects)]

____   ____   _____

Miscellaneous Compulsions

____   ____   Mental rituals (other than checking/counting)
____   ____   Excessive listmaking
____   ____   Need to tell, ask, or confess
____   ____   Need to touch, tap, or rub*
____   ____   Rituals involving blinking or staring*
____   ____   Measures (not checking) to prevent
                harm to self ____, harm to others ____, terrible
                consequences ____
____   ____   Ritualized eating behaviors*
____   ____   Superstitious behaviors
____   ____   Trichotillomania*
____   ____   Other self-damaging or self-mutilating behaviors*
____   ____   Other _____

Target symptom list

Name _____ Date _____
Obsessions

1. _____

    _____

    _____

    _____

2. _____

    _____

    _____

    _____

3. _____

    _____

    _____

    _____

Compulsions

1. _____

    _____

2. _____

3. _____

Avoidance

1. _____

2. _____

3. _____

Yale-Brown Obsessive Compulsive Scale (YBOCS)

'I am now going to ask several questions about your obsessive thoughts.' [Make specific reference to the patient's target obsessions.]

1. Time Occupied by Obsessive Thoughts

- How much of your time is occupied by obsessive thoughts? [When obsessions occur as brief, intermittent intrusions, it may be difficult to assess time occupied by them in terms of total hours. In such cases, estimate time by determining how frequently they occur. Consider both the number of times the intrusions occur and how many hours of the day are affected. Ask: How frequently do the obsessive thoughts occur? [Be sure to exclude ruminations and preoccupations, which, unlike obsessions, are ego-syntonic and rational (but exaggerated).]
0—None.
1—Mild, less than 1 hr/day or occasional intrusion
2—Moderate, 1 to 3 hr/day or frequent intrusion

3—Severe, greater than 3 and up to 8 hr/day or very frequent intrusion

4—Extreme, greater than 8 hr/day or near constant intrusion

1b. Obsession-Free Interval (not included in total score)

- On the average, what is the longest number of consecutive waking hours per day that you are completely free of obsessive thoughts? [If necessary, ask: What is the longest block of time in which obsessive thoughts are absent?]

  0—No symptoms

  1—Long symptom-free interval, more than 8 consecutive hrs/day symptom free

  2—Moderately long symptom-free interval, more than 3 and up to 8 consecutive hrs/day symptom free

  3—Short symptom-free interval, from 1 to 3 consecutive hrs/day symptom free

  4—Extremely short symptom-free interval, less than 1 consecutive hr/day symptom free

2. Interference Due to Obsessive Thoughts

- How much do your obsessive thoughts interfere with your social or work (or role) functioning? Is there anything that you don't do because of them? [If currently not working determine how much performance would be affected if patient were employed.]

  0—None

  1—Mild, slight interference with social or occupational activities, but overall performance not impaired

  2—Moderate, definite interference with social or occupational performance, but still manageable

  3—Severe, causes substantial impairment in social or occupational performance

  4—Extreme, incapacitating

3. Distress Associated with Obsessive Thoughts

- How much distress do your obsessive thoughts cause you?

  [In most cases, distress is equated with anxiety; however, patients may report that their obsessions are 'disturbing' but deny 'anxiety.' Only rate anxiety that seems triggered by obsessions, not generalized anxiety or anxiety associated with other conditions.]

  0—None

  1—Mild, not too disturbing

  2—Moderate, disturbing, but still manageable

  3—Severe, very disturbing

  4—Extreme, near constant and disabling distress

4. Resistance Against Obsessions

- How much of an effort do you make to resist the obsessive thoughts? How often do you try to disregard or turn your attention away from these thoughts as they enter your mind? [Only rate effort made to resist, not success or failure in actually controlling the obsessions. How much the patient resists the obsessions may or may not correlate with his/her ability to control them. Note that this item does not directly measure the severity of the intrusive thoughts; rather it rates a manifestation of health, i.e., the effort the patient makes to counteract the obsessions by means other than avoidance or the performance of compulsions. Thus, the more the patient tries to resist, the less impaired is this aspect of his/her functioning. There are 'active' and 'passive' forms of resistance. Patients in behavioral therapy may be encouraged to counteract their obsessive symptoms by not struggling against them (e.g., 'just let the thoughts come') passive opposition, or by intentionally bringing on the disturbing thoughts. For the purposes of this item, consider use of these behavioral techniques as forms of resistance. If the obsessions are minimal, the patient may not feel the need to resist them. In such cases, a rating of '0' should be given.]
  0—Makes an effort to always resist, or symptoms so minimal doesn't need to actively resist
  1—Tries to resist most of the time
  2—Makes some effort to resist
  3—Yields to all obsessions without attempting to control them, but does so with some reluctance
  4—Completely and willingly yields to all obsessions

5. Degree of Control over Obsessive Thoughts

- How much control do you have over your obsessive thoughts? How successful are you in stopping or diverting your obsessive thinking? Can you dismiss them? [In contrast to the preceding item on resistance, the ability of the patient to control his obsessions is more closely related to the severity of the intrusive thoughts.]
  0—Complete control
  1—Much control, usually able to stop or divert obsessions with some effort and concentration
  2—Moderate control, sometimes able to stop or divert obsessions
  3—Little control, rarely successful in stopping or dismissing obsessions, can only divert
  4—No control, experienced as completely involuntary, rarely able to even momentarily alter obsessive thinking

'The next several questions are about your compulsive behaviors.' [Make specific reference to the patient's target compulsions.]

6. Time Spent Performing Compulsive Behaviors

- How much time do you spend performing compulsive behaviors? [When rituals involving activities of daily living are chiefly present, ask: How much longer than most people does it take to complete routine activities because of your rituals? When compulsions occur as brief, intermittent behaviors, it may be difficult to assess time spent performing them in terms of total hours. In such cases, estimate time by determining how frequently they are performed. Consider both the number of times compulsions are performed and how many hours of the day are affected. Count separate occurrences of compulsive behaviors, not number of repetitions; e.g., a patient who goes into the bathroom 20 different times a day to wash his hands 5 times very quickly, performs compulsions 20 times a day, not 5 or $5 \times 20 = 100$. Ask: How frequently do you perform compulsions? In most cases compulsions are observable behaviors (e.g., hand washing), but some compulsions are covert (e.g., silent checking).]
  0—None
  1—Mild (spends less than 1 hr/day performing compulsions) or occasional performance of compulsive behaviors
  2—Moderate (spends from 1 to 3 hrs/day performing compulsions) or frequent performance of compulsive behaviors
  3—Severe (spends more than 3 and up to 8 hrs/day performing compulsions) or very frequent performance of compulsive behaviors
  4—Extreme (spends more than 8 hrs/day performing compulsions) or near constant performance of compulsive behaviors (too numerous to count)

6b. Compulsion-Free Interval (not included in total sore)

- On the average, what is the longest number of consecutive waking hours per day that you are completely free of compulsive behavior? [If necessary, ask: What is the longest block of time in which compulsions are absent?]
  0—No symptoms
  1—Long symptom-free interval, more than 8 consecutive hrs/day symptom free
  2—Moderately long symptom-free interval, more than 3 and up to 8 consecutive hrs/day symptom free
  3—Short symptom-free interval, from 1 to 3 consecutive hrs/day symptom free.
  4—Extremely short symptom-free interval, less than 1 consecutive hr/day symptom free

7. Interference due to Compulsive Behaviors

- How much do your compulsive behaviors interfere with your social or work (or role) functioning? Is there anything that you don't do because of the compulsions? [If currently not working determine how much performance would be affected if patient were employed.]
  0—None
  1—Mild, slight interference with social or occupational activities, but overall performance not impaired
  2—Moderate, definite interference with social or occupational performance, but still manageable
  3—Severe, causes substantial impairment in social or occupational performance
  4—Extreme, incapacitating

8. Distress Associated with Compulsive Behavior

- How would you feel if prevented from performing your compulsions(s)? [Pause] How anxious would you become? [Rate degree of distress patient would experience if performance of the compulsion were suddenly interrupted without reassurance offered. In most, but not all cases, performing compulsions reduces anxiety. If, in the judgment of the interviewer, anxiety is actually reduced by preventing compulsions in the manner described above, then ask: How anxious do you get while performing compulsions until you are satisfied they are completed?]
  0—None
  1—Mild only slightly anxious if compulsions prevented, or only slight anxiety during performance of compulsions
  2—Moderate, reports that anxiety would mount but remain manageable if compulsions prevented, or that anxiety increases but remains manageable during performance of compulsions
  3—Severe, prominent and very disturbing increase in anxiety if compulsions interrupted, or prominent and very disturbing increase in anxiety during performance of compulsions
  4—Extreme, incapacitating anxiety from any intervention aimed at modifying activity, or incapacitating anxiety develops during performance of compulsions

9. Resistance Against Compulsions

- How much of an effort do you make to resist the compulsions? [Only rate effort made to resist, not success or failure in actually controlling the compulsions. How much the patient resists the compulsions may or may not correlate with his ability to control them. Note that this item does not directly measure the severity of the compulsions; rather it rates a manifestation of health, i.e., the effort the patient makes to counteract the compulsions. Thus, the more the patient tries to resist, the less impaired is this aspect of his functioning. If the compulsions are minimal, the patient may not feel the need to resist them. In such cases, a rating of '0' should be given.]

0—Makes an effort to always resist, or symptoms so minimal doesn't need to actively resist

1—Tries to resist most of the time

2—Makes some effort to resist

3—Yields to almost all compulsions without attempting to control them, but does so with some reluctance

4—Completely and willingly yields to all compulsions

10. Degree of Control over Compulsive Behavior

• How strong is the drive to perform the compulsive behavior? [Pause] How much control do you have over the compulsions? [In contrast to the preceding item on resistance, the ability of the patient to control his compulsions is more closely related to the severity of the compulsions.]

0—Complete control

1—Much control, experiences pressure to perform the behavior but usually able to exercise voluntary control over it

2—Moderate control, strong pressure to perform behavior, can control it only with difficulty

3—Little control, very strong drive to perform behavior, must be carried to completion, can only delay with difficulty

4—No control, drive to perform behavior experienced as completely involuntary and overpowering, rarely able to even momentarily delay activity

'The remaining questions are about both obsessions and compulsions. Some ask about related problems.' These are investigational items not included in total YBOCS score but may be useful in assessing these symptoms.

11. Insight into Obsessions and Compulsions

• Do you think your concerns or behaviors are reasonable? [Pause] What do you think would happen if you did not perform the compulsion(s)? Are you convinced something would really happen? [Rate patient's insight into the senselessness or excessiveness of his obsession(s) based on beliefs expressed at the time of the interview.]

0—Excellent insight, fully rational

1—Good insight. Readily acknowledges absurdity or excessiveness of thoughts or behaviors but does not seem completely convinced that there isn't something besides anxiety to be concerned about (i.e., has lingering doubts)

2—Fair insight. Reluctantly admits thoughts or behavior seem unreasonable or excessive, but wavers. May have some unrealistic fears, but no fixed convictions

3—Poor insight. Maintains that thoughts or behaviors are not unreasonable or excessive, but acknowledges validity of contrary evidence (i.e., overvalued ideas present)

4—Lacks insight, delusional. Definitely convinced that concerns and behavior are reasonable, unresponsive to contrary evidence

12. Avoidance

• Have you been avoiding doing anything, going any place, or being with anyone because of your obsessional thoughts or out of concern you will perform compulsions? [If yes, then ask: How much do you avoid? Rate degree to which patient deliberately tries to avoid things. Sometimes compulsions are designed to 'avoid' contact with something that the patient fears. For example, clothes washing rituals would be designated as compulsions, not as avoidant behavior. If the patient stopped doing the laundry then this would constitute avoidance.]

0—No deliberate avoidance

1—Mild, minimal avoidance

2—Moderate, some avoidance; clearly present

3—Severe, much avoidance; avoidance prominent

4—Extreme, very extensive avoidance; patient does almost everything he/she can to avoid triggering symptoms

13. Degree of Indecisiveness

• Do you have trouble making decisions about little things that other people might not think twice about (e.g., which clothes to put on in the morning; which brand of cereal to buy)? [Exclude difficulty making decisions which reflect ruminative thinking. Ambivalence concerning rationally-based difficult choices should also be excluded.]

0—None

1—Mild, some trouble making decisions about minor things

2—Moderate, freely reports significant trouble making decisions that others would not think twice about

3—Severe, continual weighing of pros and cons about nonessentials

4—Extreme, unable to make any decisions. Disabling

14. Overvalued Sense of Responsibility

• Do you feel very responsible for the consequences of your actions? Do you blame yourself for the outcome of events not completely in your control? [Distinguish from normal feelings of responsibility, feelings of worthlessness, and pathological guilt. A guilt-ridden person experiences himself or his actions as bad or evil.]

0—None

1—Mild, only mentioned on questioning, slight sense of over-responsibility

2—Moderate, ideas stated spontaneously, clearly present; patient experiences significant sense of over-responsibility for events outside his/her reasonable control

3—Severe, ideas prominent and pervasive; deeply concerned he/she is responsible for events clearly outside his control. Self-blaming farfetched and nearly irrational

4—Extreme, delusional sense of responsibility (e.g., if an earthquake occurs 3,000 miles away patient blames herself because she didn't perform her compulsions)

15. Pervasive Slowness/Disturbance of Inertia

• Do you have difficulty starting or finishing tasks? Do many routine activities take longer than they should? [Distinguish from psychomotor retardation secondary to depression. Rate increased time spent performing routine activities even when specific obsessions cannot be identified.]

0—None

1—Mild, occasional delay in starting or finishing

2—Moderate, frequent prolongation of routine activities but tasks usually completed. Frequently late

3—Severe, pervasive and marked difficulty initiating and completing routine tasks. Usually late

4—Extreme, unable to start or complete routine tasks without full assistance

16. Pathological Doubting

• After you complete an activity do you doubt whether you performed it correctly? Do you doubt whether you did it at all? When carrying out routine activities do you find that you don't trust your senses (i.e., what you see, hear, or touch)?

0—None

1—Mild, only mentioned on questioning, slight pathological doubt. Examples given may be within normal range

2—Moderate, ideas stated spontaneously, clearly present and apparent in some of patient's behaviors; patient bothered by significant pathological doubt. Some effect on performance but still manageable

3—Severe, uncertainty about perceptions or memory prominent; pathological doubt frequently affects performance

4—Extreme, uncertainty about perceptions constantly present; pathological doubt substantially affects almost all activities. Incapacitating (e.g., patient states 'my mind doesn't trust what my eyes see')

[Items 17 and 18 refer to global illness severity. The rater is required to consider global function, not just the severity of obsessive-compulsive symptoms.]

17. Global Severity

Interviewer's judgment of the overall severity of the patient's illness. Rated from 0 (no illness) to 6 (most severe patient seen). [Consider the degree of distress reported by the patient, the symptoms observed, and the functional impairment reported. Your judgment is required both in averaging this data as well as weighing the reliability or accuracy of the data obtained. This judgment is based on information obtained during the interview.]

0—No illness

1—Illness slight, doubtful, transient; no functional impairment

2—Mild symptoms, little functional impairment

3—Moderate symptoms, functions with effort

4—Moderate – severe symptoms, limited functioning

5—Severe symptoms, functions mainly with assistance

6—Extremely severe symptoms, completely nonfunctional

18. Global Improvement

Rate total overall improvement present *since the initial rating*, whether or not, in your judgment, it is due to drug treatment.

0—Very much worse

1—Much worse

2—Minimally worse

3—No change

4—Minimally improved

5—Much improved

6—Very much improved

19. Reliability

Rate the overall reliability of the rating scores obtained. Factors that may affect reliability include the patient's cooperativeness and his/her natural ability to communicate. The type and severity of obsessive-compulsive symptoms present may interfere with the patient's concentration, attention, or freedom to speak spontaneously (e.g., the content of some obsessions may cause the patient to choose his words very carefully).

0—Excellent, no reason to suspect data unreliable

1—Good, factor(s) present that may adversely affect reliability

2—Fair, factor(s) present that definitely reduce reliability

3—Poor, very low reliability

Items 17 and 18 are adapted from the Clinical Global Impression Scale (Guy W: ECDEU Assessment Manual for Psychopharmacology: Publication 76-338. Washington, DC, US Department of Health, Education, and Welfare, 1976).

Additional information regarding the development, use, and psychometric properties of the YBOCS can be found in Goodman WK, Price LH, Rasmussen SA, et al: The Yale–Brown Obsessive Compulsive Scale (YBOCS). Part I: Development, use, and reliability. *Arch Gen Psychiatry* (1989) **46**:1006–11, and Goodman WK, Price LH, Rasmussen SA, et al: The Yale–Brown Obsessive Compulsive Scale (YBOCS). Part II: Validity. *Arch Gen Psychiatry* (1989) **46**:1012–16.

Yale–Brown Obsessive Compulsive Scale (9/89)

YBOCS total (add items 1–10) ☐
Patient name _____
Patient ID _____
Date _____
Rater _____

		None	Mild	Moderate	Severe	Extreme
1.	Time spent on obsessions	0	1	2	3	4

1b. Obsession-free interval	No Symptoms	Long	Moderately Long	Short	Extremely Short
(do not add to subtotal or total score)	0	1	2	3	4

2.	Interference from obsessions	0	1	2	3	4
3.	Distress of obsessions	0	1	2	3	4
		Always Resists				Completely Yields
4.	Resistance	0	1	2	3	4
		Complete Control	Much Control	Moderate Control	Little Control	No Control
5.	Control over obsessions	0	1	2	3	4

Obsession subtotal (add items 1–5) ☐

		None	Mild	Moderate	Severe	Extreme
6.	Time spent on compulsions	0	1	2	3	4

6b. Compulsion-free interval	No Symptoms	Long	Moderately Long	Short	Extremely Short
(do not add to subtotal or total score)	0	1	2	3	4

7.	Interference from compulsions	0	1	2	3	4
8.	Distress from compulsions	0	1	2	3	4
		Always Resists				Completely Yields
9.	Resistance	0	1	2	3	4
		Complete Control	Much Control	Moderate Control	Little Control	No Control
10.	Control over compulsions	0	1	2	3	4

Compulsion subtotal (add items 6–10) ☐

		Excellent				Absent
11.	Insight into O-C symptoms	0	1	2	3	4

		None	Mild	Moderate	Severe	Extreme
12.	Avoidance	0	1	2	3	4
13.	Indecisiveness	0	1	2	3	4
14.	Pathologic responsibility	0	1	2	3	4
15.	Slowness	0	1	2	3	4
16.	Pathologic doubting	0	1	2	3	4

17.	Global severity	0	1	2	3	4	5	6
18.	Global improvement	0	1	2	3	4	5	6

19.	Reliability:	Excellent = 0	Good = 1	Fair = 2	Poor = 3

Childrens' Yale–Brown Obsessive Compulsive Scale (CY–BOCS)

Developed by Wayne K Goodman, MD, Steven A Rasmussen, MD, Mark A Riddle, MD, Lawrence H Price, MD, Judith L Rapoport, MD, of the Department of Psychiatry, University of Florida College of Medicine; Department of Psychiatry, Johns Hopkins University School of Medicine; Department of Psychiatry, Brown University School of Medicine; Department of Psychiatry, Yale University School of Medicine; and Child Psychiatric Branch, National Institute of Mental Health.

Investigators interested in using this rating scale should contact Dr Goodman at the University of Florida, Department of Psychiatry, PO Box 100256, Gainesville, FL 32610.

Copyright Wayne K Goodman, MD, 1989. Reproduced with permission.

General instructions

Overview

This scale is designed to rate the severity of obsessive and compulsive symptoms in children, ages 6 to 17 years. In general, the ratings depend on the child's and parent's report, however, the final rating is based on the clinical judgment of the interviewer. Rate the characteristics of each item during the prior week up until and including the time of the interview. Scores should reflect the average (mean) occurrence of each item for the entire week, unless specified otherwise.

Informants

Ideally, information should be obtained by interviewing: (1) the parent(s) or guardian alone, (2) the child alone and, (3) the child and parent(s) together (to clarify differences). The preferred order for the interviews may vary depending on the age and developmental level of the child or adolescent. Information from each of these interviews should then be combined to inform the scoring of each item. Consistent reporting can be ensured by having the *same informant(s) present for each rating session.*

Definitions

Before proceeding with the questions, define 'obsessions' and 'compulsions' for the child and primary caretaker as follows:
'*Obsessions* are thoughts, ideas, or pictures that keep coming into your mind even though you do not want them to. They may be unpleasant, silly or embarrassing.'

'*An example of an obsession is* the repeated thought that germs or dirt are harming you or other people, or that something unpleasant may happen to your or someone special to you.' These are thoughts that keep coming back, over and over again.

'*Compulsions* are things that you feel you have to do although you may know that they do not make sense. Sometimes, you may try to stop from doing them but this might not be possible. You might feel worried or angry or frustrated until you have finished what you have to do.'

'*An example of a compulsion is* the need to wash your hands over and over again even though they are not really dirty, or the need to count up to a certain number while you do certain things.'

'Do you have any questions about what these words called compulsions and obsessions mean?'

Symptom specificity

The rater must determine that reported behaviors are true obsessions or compulsions and not other symptoms, such as phobias or anxious worries. The differential diagnosis between certain complex motor tics and certain compulsions (e.g. touching or tapping) may be difficult or impossible. In such cases, it is particularly important to provide explicit descriptions of the target symptoms and to be consistent in including or excluding these symptoms in subsequent ratings. Separate assessment of tic severity with a tic rating instrument may be necessary in such cases.

Some of the items listed on the CY–BOCS Symptom Checklist, such as trichotillomania, are currently classified in DSM-III-R as symptoms of an Impulse Control Disorder.

Items marked '*' in the Symptom Checklist may or may not be obsessions or compulsions.

Procedure

This scale is designed to be used by a clinician in a *semi-structured interview format.* After reviewing with the child and parent(s) the definitions of obsessions and compulsions, inquire about specific compulsions and complete the CY–BOCS Compulsions Checklist on pages 24–5. Then complete the Target Symptom List for Compulsions on page 26. Next, inquire about and note questions 6 through 10 on pages 26 through 29, repeat the above procedure for obsessions: review definitions, complete the Obsessions Checklist on pages 20–2, complete the Target Symptom List for obsessions on page 21–2, and inquire about and rate questions 1 through 5 on pages 22–4.

Finally, inquire about and rate questions 11 through 19 on pages 29 through 32. Scoring can be recorded on the scoring sheet on page 33. All ratings should be in whole integers.

Scoring

All 19 items are rated, but only items 1–10 are used to determine the total score. The total CY–BOCS score is the sum of items 1–10, whereas the obsession and compulsion subtotals are the sums of items 1–5 and 6–10, respectively. 1B and 6B are not being used in the scoring.

Items 17 (global severity) and 18 (global improvement) are adapted from the Clinical Global Impression Scale (Guy W, 1976: ECDEU Assessment Manual for Psychopharmacology: Publication 76–338. Washington, DC, US Department of Health, Education, and Welfare, 1976.) to provide measures of overall functional impairment associated with the presence of obsessive-compulsive symptoms.

Name _____ Date _____

CY-BOCS obsessions checklist

Check all that apply, but clearly mark the principal symptoms with a 'P'. (Item marked '*' may or may not be OCD phenomena.)

Current	Past	
		Contamination Obsessions
____	____	Concern with dirt, germs, certain illnesses (e.g., AIDS)
____	____	Concern or disgust with bodily waste or secretions (e.g., urine, feces, saliva)
____	____	Excessive concern with environmental contaminants (e.g., asbestos, radiation, toxic waste)
____	____	Excessive concern with household items (e.g., cleaners, solvents)
____	____	Excessive concern about animals/insects
____	____	Excessively bothered by sticky substances or residues
____	____	Concerned will get ill because of contaminant
____	____	Concerned will get others ill by spreading contaminant (aggressive)
____	____	No concern with consequences of contamination other than how it might feel*
____	____	Other (describe) _____
		Aggressive Obsessions
____	____	Fear might harm self
____	____	Fear might harm others
____	____	Fear harm will come to self
____	____	Fear harm will come to others because something child did or did not do
____	____	Violent or horrific images
____	____	Fear of blurting out obscenities or insults
____	____	Fear of doing something else embarrassing*

_____ _____ Fear will act on unwanted impulses (e.g., to stab a family
member)

_____ _____ Fear will steal things

_____ _____ Fear will be responsible for something else terrible happening
(e.g., fire, burglary, flood)

_____ _____ Other (describe) _____

Sexual Obsessions
(Are you having any sexual thoughts? If yes, are they routine or
are they repetitive thoughts that you would rather not have or
find disturbing? If yes, are they:)

_____ _____ Forbidden or perverse sexual thoughts, images, impulses

_____ _____ Content involves homosexuality*

_____ _____ Sexual behavior toward others (aggressive)*

_____ _____ Other (describe) _____

Hoarding/Saving Obsessions

_____ _____ Fear of losing things

Magical Thoughts/ Superstitious Obsessions

_____ _____ Lucky/unlucky numbers

_____ _____ Other (describe) _____

Somatic Obsessions

_____ _____ Excessive concern with illness or disease*

_____ _____ Excessive concern with body part or aspect of appearance
(e.g., dysmorphophobia)*

Religious Obsessions

_____ _____ Excessive concern or fear of offending religious objects (God)

_____ _____ Excess concern with right/wrong, morality

_____ _____ Other (describe) _____

Miscellaneous Obsessions

_____ _____ Need to know or remember

_____ _____ Fear of saying certain things

_____ _____ Fear of not saying just the right thing

_____ _____ Intrusive (non-violent) images

_____ _____ Intrusive sounds, words, music, or numbers

_____ _____ Other (describe) _____

Target symptom list for obsessions

Obsessions (Describe, listing by order of severity):

1. _____

   _____

2. _____

   _____

3. _____

   _____

4.   _____
     _____

Avoidance (Describe any avoidance behavior associated with obsessions; e.g., child *avoids* putting clothes away to prevent thoughts.)

_____
_____
_____
_____

Questions on obsessions (items 1–5)

'I am now going to ask you questions about the thoughts you cannot stop thinking about.'

1. Time Occupied by Obsessive Thoughts

- How much time do you spend thinking about these things?
  (When obsessions occur as brief, intermittent intrusions, it may be impossible to assess time occupied by them in terms of total hours. In such cases, estimate time by determining how frequently they occur. Consider both the number of times the intrusions occur and how many hours of the day are affected.)

- How frequently do these thoughts occur?
  (Be sure to exclude ruminations and preoccupations which, unlike obsessions, are ego-syntonic and rational [but exaggerated].)
  0—None
  1—Mild, less than 1 hr/day or occasional intrusion
  2—Moderate, 1 to 3 hrs/day or frequent intrusion
  3—Severe, greater than 3 and up to 8 hrs/day or very frequent intrusion
  4—Extreme, greater than 8 hrs/day or near constant intrusion

1b. Obsession-Free Interval (not included in total score)

- On the average, what is the longest amount of time each day that you are not bothered by the obsessive thoughts?
  0—None
  1—Mild, long symptom free intervals or more than 8 consecutive hrs/day symptom-free
  2—Moderate, moderately long symptom-free intervals or more than 3 and up to 8 consecutive hrs/day symptom-free

3—Severe, brief symptom-free intervals or from 1 to 3 consecutive hrs/day symptom-free

4—Extreme, less than 1 consecutive hr/day symptom-free

2. Interference due to Obsessive Thoughts

• How much do these thoughts get in the way of school or doing things with friends?

• Is there anything that you don't do because of them?
(If currently not in school determine how much performance would be affected if patient were in school.)
0—None
1—Mild, slight interference with social or school activities, but overall performance not impaired
2—Moderate, definite interference with social or school performance, but still manageable
3—Severe, causes substantial impairment in social or school performance
4—Extreme, incapacitating

3. Distress Associated with Obsessive Thoughts

• How much do these thoughts bother or upset you?
(Only rate anxiety/frustration that seems triggered by obsessions, not generalized anxiety or anxiety associated with other symptoms.)
0—None
1—Mild, infrequent, and not too disturbing
2—Moderate, frequent, and disturbing, but still manageable
3—Severe, very frequent, and very disturbing
4—Extreme, near constant, and disabling distress/frustration

4. Resistance against Obsessions

• How hard do you try to stop the thoughts or ignore them?
(Only rate effort made to resist, not success or failure in actually controlling the obsessions. How much patient resists the obsessions may or may not correlate with their ability to control them. Note that this item does not directly measure the severity of the intrusive thoughts; rather it rates a manifestation of health, i.e., the effort the patient makes to counteract the obsessions. Thus, the more the patient tries to resist, the less impaired is this aspect of his/her functioning. If the obsessions are minimal, the patient may not feel the need to resist them. In such cases, a rating of '0' should be given.)
0—None, makes an effort to always resist or symptoms so minimal doesn't need to actively resist

1—Mild, tries to resist most of the time

2—Moderate, makes some effort to resist

3—Severe, yields to all obsessions without attempting to control them, but does so with some reluctance

4—Extreme, completely and willingly yields to all obsessions

5. Degree of Control over Obsessive Thoughts

• When you try to fight the thoughts, can you beat them?

• How much control do you have over the thoughts?
(In contrast to the preceding item on resistance, the ability of the patient to control his/her obsessions is more closely related to the severity of the intrusive thoughts.)

0—Complete control

1—Much control, usually able to stop or divert obsessions with some effort and concentration

2—Moderate control, sometimes able to stop or divert obsessions

3—Little control, rarely successful in stopping obsessions, can only divert attention with difficulty

4—No control, experienced as completely involuntary, rarely able to even momentarily divert thinking

Name _____ Date _____

CY–BOCS Compulsions Checklist

Check all that apply, but clearly mark the principal symptoms with a 'P'. (Items marked '*' may or may not be compulsions.)

Current	Past	*Washing/Cleaning Compulsions*
____	____	Excessive or ritualized handwashing
____	____	Excessive or ritualized showering, bathing, toothbrushing, grooming, or toilet routine
____	____	Excessive cleaning of items (e.g. personal clothes or important items)
____	____	Other measures to prevent or remove contact with contaminants
____	____	Other (describe) _____

Current	Past	*Checking Compulsions*
____	____	Checking locks, toys, school books/items, etc.
____	____	Checking associated with getting washed, dressed, or undressed
____	____	Checking that did not/will not harm others
____	____	Checking that did not/will not harm self
____	____	Checking that nothing terrible did/will happen

____ ____ Checking that did not make mistake
____ ____ Checking tied to somatic obsessions
____ ____ Other (describe) _____

Repeating Compulsions
____ ____ Rereading, erasing, or rewriting
____ ____ Need to repeat routine activities (e.g., in/out door, up/down
            from chair)
____ ____ Other (describe) _____

Counting Compulsions
            Objects, certain numbers, words, etc.
____ ____ Other (describe) _____

Ordering/Arranging Compulsions
            Need for symmetry or evening up (e.g., lining items up a certain
            way or arranging personal items in specific patterns)
____ ____ Other (describe) _____

Hoarding/Saving Compulsions
            (distinguish from hobbies and concern with objects of monetary
            or sentimental value)
____ ____ Difficulty throwing things away, saving bits of paper, string, etc.
____ ____ Other (describe) _____

Excessive Magical Games/Superstitious Behaviors
            (distinguish from age appropriate magical games)
            (e.g., array of behavior, such as stepping over certain spots on
            a floor, touching an object/self certain number of times as a
            routine game to avoid something bad from happening.)
____ ____ Other (describe) _____

Rituals Involving Other Persons
            The need to involve another person (usually a parent) in ritual
            (e.g., asking a parent to repeatedly answer the same questions,
            making parent perform certain meal time rituals involving
            specific utensils.*)
____ ____ Describe _____

Miscellaneous Compulsions
____ ____ Mental rituals (other than counting)
____ ____ Need to tell, ask, confess
____ ____ Measures (not checking) to prevent:
            harm to self ____; harm to others ____; terrible consequences
            ____
____ ____ Ritualized eating behaviors*
____ ____ Excessive list making*
____ ____ Need to touch, tap, rub
____ ____ Need to do things (e.g., touch or arrange) until it *feels* just right*
____ ____ Rituals involving blinking or staring*
____ ____ Trichotillomania (hair pulling)*
____ ____ Other self-damaging or self-mutilating behavior*
____ ____ Other (describe) _____

Target symptom list for compulsions

Compulsions (Describe, listing by order of severity):

1. _____

_____

2. _____

_____

3. _____

_____

4. _____

_____

Avoidance (Describe any avoidance behavior associated with compulsions; e.g., child *avoids* putting clothes away to prevent start of counting behavior.)

_____

_____

_____

Questions on compulsions (items 6–10)

'I am now going to ask you questions about the habits you can't stop.'

6a. Time Spent Performing Compulsive Behaviors

- How much time do you spend doing these things?
- How much longer than most people does it take to complete your usual daily activities because of the habits?
  (When compulsions occur as brief, intermittent behaviors, it may be impossible to assess time spent performing them in terms of total hours. In such cases, estimate time by determining how frequently they are performed. Consider both the number of times compulsions are performed and how many hours of the day are affected.)
- How often do you do these habits?
  [In most cases compulsions are observable behaviors (e.g., hand-washing), but there are instances in which compulsions are not observable (e.g., silent checking).]
  0—None
  1—Mild, spends less than 1 hr/day performing compulsions or occasional performance of compulsive behaviors
  2—Moderate, spends from 1 to 3 hrs/day performing compulsions or frequent performance of compulsive behaviors
  3—Severe, spends more than 3 and up to 8 hrs/day performing compulsions or very frequent performance of compulsive behaviors

4—Extreme, spends more than 8 hrs/day performing compulsions or near constant performance of compulsive behaviors

6b. Compulsion-Free Interval

- How long can you go without performing compulsive behavior?
  [If necessary ask: What is the longest block of time in which (your habits) compulsions are absent?]
  0—No symptoms
  1—Mild, long symptom-free interval or more than 8 consecutive hrs/day symptom-free
  2—Moderate, moderately long symptom-free interval or more than 3 and up to 8 consecutive hrs/day symptom-free
  3—Severe, short symptom-free interval or from 1 to 3 consecutive hrs/day symptom-free
  4—Extreme, less than 1 consecutive hr/day symptom-free

7. Interference due to Compulsive Behaviors

- How much do these habits get in the way of school or doing things with friends?
- Is there anything you don't do because of them?
  (If currently not in school, determine how much performance would be affected if patient were in school.)
  0—None
  1—Mild, slight interference with social or school activities, but overall performance not impaired
  2—Moderate, definite interference with social or school performance, but still manageable
  3—Severe, causes substantial impairment in social or school performance
  4—Extreme, incapacitating

8. Distress Associated with Compulsive Behavior

- How would you feel if prevented from carrying out your habits?
- How upset would you become?
  (Rate degree of distress/frustration patient would experience if performance of the compulsion were suddenly interrupted without reassurance offered. In most, but not all cases, performing compulsions reduces anxiety/frustration.)
- How upset do you get while carrying out your habits until you are satisfied?
  0—None
  1—Mild, only slightly anxious/frustrated if compulsions prevented; only slight anxiety/frustration during performance of compulsions

2—Moderate, reports that anxiety/frustration would mount but remain manageable if compulsions prevented; anxiety/frustration increases but remains manageable during performance of compulsions

3—Severe, prominent and very disturbing increase in anxiety/frustration if compulsions interrupted; prominent and very disturbing increase in anxiety/frustration during performance of compulsions

4—Extreme, incapacitating anxiety/frustration from any intervention aimed at modifying activity; incapacitating anxiety/frustration develops during performance of compulsions

9. Resistance against Compulsions

- How much do you try to fight the habits?

(Only rate effort made to resist, not success or failure in actually controlling the compulsions. How much the patient resists the compulsions may or may not correlate with his/her ability to control them. Note that this item does not directly measure the severity of the compulsions, rather it rates a manifestation of health, i.e. the effort the patient makes to counteract the compulsions. Thus, the more the patient tries to resist, the less impaired is this aspect of his/her functioning. If the compulsions are minimal, the patient may not feel the need to resist them. In such cases, a rating of '0' should be given.)

0—None, makes an effort to always resist or symptoms so minimal doesn't need to actively resist

1—Mild, tries to resist most of the time

2—Moderate, makes some effort to resist

3—Severe, yields to almost all compulsions without attempting to control them, but does so with some reluctance

4—Extreme, completely and willingly yields to all compulsions

10. Degree of Control over Compulsive Behavior

- How strong is the feeling that you have to carry out the habit(s)?
- When you try to fight them what happens?

(For the advanced child ask:)

- How much control do you have over the habits?

(In contrast to the preceding item on resistance, the ability of the patient to control his/her compulsions is closely related to the severity of the compulsions.)

0—Complete control

1—Much control, experiences pressure to perform the behavior, but usually able to exercise voluntary control over it

2—Moderate control, moderate control, strong pressure to perform behavior, can control it only with difficulty

3—Little control, little control, very strong drive to perform behavior, must be carried to completion, can only delay with difficulty

4—No control, no control, drive to perform behavior experienced as completely involuntary and overpowering, rarely able to even momentarily delay activity

11. Insight into Obsessions and Compulsions

- Do you think your concerns or behaviors are reasonable? (Pause)
- What do you think would happen if you did not perform the compulsion(s)?
- Are you convinced something would really happen?
  (Rate patient's insight into the senselessness or excessiveness of his/her obsession(s) or compulsion(s) based on beliefs expressed at the time of the interview.)
  0—None, excellent insight, fully rational
  1—Mild, good insight, readily acknowledges absurdity or excessiveness of thoughts or behaviors but does not seem completely convinced that there isn't something besides anxiety to be concerned about (i.e., has lingering doubts)
  2—Moderate, fair insight, reluctantly admits thoughts or behavior seem unreasonable or excessive, but wavers; may have some unrealistic fears, but no fixed convictions
  3—Severe, poor insight, maintains that thoughts or behaviors are not reasonable or excessive, but wavers; may have some unrealistic fears, but acknowledges validity of contrary evidence (i.e., overvalued ideas present)
  4—Extreme, lacks insight, delusional, definitely convinced that concerns and behavior are reasonable, unresponsive to contrary evidence

12. Avoidance

- Have you been avoiding doing anything, going any place, or being with anyone because of your obsessional thoughts or out of concern you will perform compulsions? (If yes, then ask:)
- How much do you avoid? (note what is avoided on symptom list)
  (Rate degree to which patient deliberately tries to avoid things. Sometimes compulsions are designed to 'avoid' contact with something that the patient fears. For example, excessive washing of fruits and vegetables to remove 'germs' would be designated as a compulsion not as an avoidant behavior. If the patient stopped eating fruits and vegetables, then this would constitute avoidance.)
  0—None
  1—Mild, minimal avoidance
  2—Moderate, some avoidance clearly present
  3—Severe, much avoidance; avoidance prominent
  4—Extreme, very extensive avoidance, patient does almost everything he/she can to avoid triggering symptoms

13. Degree of Indecisiveness

- Do you have trouble making decisions about little things that other people might not think twice about (e.g., which clothes to put on in the morning, which brand of cereal to buy)?
  (Exclude difficulty making decisions which reflect ruminative thinking. Ambivalence concerning rationally-based difficult choices should also be excluded.)
  0—None
  1—Mild, some trouble making decisions about minor things
  2—Moderate, freely reports significant trouble making decisions that others would not think twice about
  3—Severe, continual weighing of pros and cons about nonessentials
  4—Extreme, unable to make any decisions, disabling

14. Overvalued Sense of Responsibility

- Do you feel overly responsible for what you do and what effect this has on things?
- Do you blame yourself for the things that are not within your control?
  (Distinguish from normal feelings of responsibility, feelings of worthlessness, and pathological guilt. A guilt-ridden person experiences him/herself or his/her actions as bad or evil.)
  0—None
  1—Mild, only mentioned on questioning, slight sense of over responsibility
  2—Moderate, ideas stated spontaneously, clearly present, patient experiences significant sense of over-responsibility for events outside his/her reasonable control
  3—Severe, ideas prominent and pervasive, deeply concerned he/she is responsible for events clearly outside his control, self-blaming farfetched and nearly irrational
  4—Extreme, delusional sense of responsibility (e.g., if an earthquake occurs 3,000 miles away patient blames themselves because they didn't perform their compulsions)

15. Pervasive Slowness/Disturbance of Inertia

- Do you have difficulty starting or finishing tasks?
- Do many routine activities take longer than they should?
  (Distinguish from psychomotor retardation secondary to depression. Rate increased time spent performing routine activities even when specific obsessions cannot be identified.)
  0—None
  1—Mild, occasional delay in starting or finishing tasks/activities

2—Moderate, frequent prolongation of routine activities but tasks usually completed, frequently late

3—Severe, pervasive and marked difficulty initiating and completing routine tasks, usually late

4—Extreme, unable to start or complete routine tasks without full assistance

16. Pathological Doubting

- When you complete an activity do you doubt whether you performed it correctly?
- Do you doubt whether you did it at all?
- When carrying out routine activities do you find that you don't trust your senses (i.e. what you see, hear, or touch)?

0—None

1—Mild, only mentioned on questioning, slight pathological doubt, examples given may be within normal range

2—Moderate, ideas stated spontaneously, clearly present and apparent in some of patient's behaviors, patient bothered by significant pathological doubt; some effect on performance but still manageable

3—Severe, uncertainty about perceptions or memory prominent; pathological doubt frequently affects performance

4—Extreme, uncertainty about perceptions constantly present; pathological doubt substantially affects almost all activities, incapacitating (e.g., patient states 'my mind doesn't trust what my eyes see')

17. Global Severity

- Interviewer's judgement of the overall severity of the patient's illness.
- Rated from 0 (no illness) to 6 (most severe patient seen).

(Consider the degree of distress reported by the patient, the symptoms observed, and the functional impairment reported. Your judgement is required both in averaging this data as well as weighing the reliability or accuracy of the data obtained. This judgement is based on information obtained during the interview.)

0—No illness

1—Slight, illness slight, doubtful, or transient; no functional impairment

2—Mild, little functional impairment

3—Moderate, functions with effort

4—Moderate–severe, limited functioning

5—Severe, functions mainly with assistance

6—Extremely severe, completely nonfunctional

18. Global Improvement

- Rate total overall improvement present *since the initial rating* whether or not, in your judgement, it is due to drug treatment.
  0—Very much worse
  1—Much worse
  2—Minimally worse
  3—No change
  4—Minimally improved
  5—Much improved
  6—Very much improved

19. Reliability

Rate the overall reliability of the rating scores obtained. Factors that may affect reliability include the patient's cooperativeness and his/her natural ability to communicate. The type and severity of obsessive-compulsive symptoms present may interfere with the patient's concentration, attention, or freedom to speak spontaneously (e.g., the content of some obsessions may cause the patient to choose his/her words very carefully).
0—Excellent, no reason to suspect data unreliable
1—Good, factor(s) present that may adversely affect reliability
2—Fair, factor(s) present that definitely reduce reliability
3—Poor, very low reliability

Children's Yale–Brown Obsessive Compulsive Scale (3/1/90)

Patient name _____

Patient ID _____

CY–BOCS total (add items 1–10) ☐

Date _____

Rater _____

		None	**Mild**	**Moderate**	**Severe**	**Extreme**
1.	Time spent on obsessions	0	1	2	3	4

1b. Obsession-free interval	No Symptoms	Long	Moderately Long	Short	Extremely Short
(do not add to subtotal or total score)	0	1	2	3	4

		None	Mild	Moderate	Severe	Extreme
2.	Interference from obsessions	0	1	2	3	4
3.	Distress of obsessions	0	1	2	3	4
		Always Resists				Completely Yields
4.	Resistance	0	1	2	3	4
		Complete Control	Much Control	Moderate Control	Little Control	No Control
5.	Control over obsessions	0	1	2	3	4

Obsession subtotal (add items 1–5) ☐

		None	**Mild**	**Moderate**	**Severe**	**Extreme**
6.	Time spent on compulsions	0	1	2	3	4

6b. Compulsion-free interval	No Symptoms	Long	Moderately Long	Short	Extremely Short
(do not add to subtotal or total score)	0	1	2	3	4

		None	Mild	Moderate	Severe	Extreme
7.	Interference from compulsions	0	1	2	3	4
8.	Distress from compulsions	0	1	2	3	4
		Always Resists				Completely Yields
9.	Resistance	0	1	2	3	4
		Complete Control	Much Control	Moderate Control	Little Control	No Control
10.	Control over compulsions	0	1	2	3	4

Compulsion subtotal (add items 6–10) ☐

		Excellent				Absent
11.	Insight into O-C symptoms	0	1	2	3	4

		None	**Mild**	**Moderate**	**Severe**	**Extreme**
12.	Avoidance	0	1	2	3	4
13.	Indecisiveness	0	1	2	3	4
14.	Pathologic responsibility	0	1	2	3	4
15.	Slowness	0	1	2	3	4
16.	Pathologic doubting	0	1	2	3	4

17.	Global severity	0	1	2	3	4	5	6
18.	Global improvement	0	1	2	3	4	5	6

19.	Reliability:	Excellent = 0	Good = 1	Fair = 2	Poor = 3

Maudsley Obsessive-Compulsive Inventory*

Name _____   Date _____

INSTRUCTIONS: Please answer each question by putting a circle around the '*True*' or the '*False*' following the question. There are no right or wrong answers and no trick questions. Work quickly and do not think about the exact meaning of the question.†

1.	I avoid using public telephones because of possible contamination.	*True*	False
2.	I frequently get nasty thoughts and have difficulty in getting rid of them.	*True*	False
3.	I am more concerned than most people about honesty.	*True*	False
4.	I am often late because I can't seem to get through everything on time.	*True*	False
5.	I don't worry unduly about contamination if I touch an animal.	True	*False*
6.	I frequently have to check things (e.g., gas or water taps, doors) several times.	*True*	False
7.	I have a very strict conscience.	*True*	False
8.	I find that almost every day I am upset by unpleasant thoughts that come into my mind against my will.	*True*	False
9.	I do not worry unduly if I accidentally bump into somebody.	True	*False*
10.	I usually have serious doubts about the simple everyday things I do.	*True*	False
11.	Neither of my parents was very strict during my childhood.	True	*False*
12.	I tend to get behind in my work because I repeat things over and over again.	*True*	False
13.	I use only an average amount of soap.	True	*False*
14.	Some numbers are extremely unlucky.	*True*	False
15.	I do not check letters over and over again before mailing them.	True	*False*
16.	I do not take a long time to dress in the morning.	True	*False*
17.	I am not excessively concerned about cleanliness.	True	*False*
18.	One of my major problems is that I pay too much attention to detail.	*True*	False
19.	I can use well-kept toilets without any hesitation.	True	*False*
20.	My major problem is repeated checking.	*True*	False
21.	I am not unduly concerned about germs and diseases.	True	*False*
22.	I do not tend to check things more than once.	True	*False*
23.	I do not stick to a very strict routine when doing ordinary things.	True	*False*
24.	My hands do not feel dirty after touching money.	True	*False*
25.	I do not usually count when doing a routine task.	True	*False*
26.	I take rather a long time to complete my washing in the morning.	*True*	False
27.	I do not use a great deal of antiseptics.	True	*False*

*Reprinted from *Behav Res Ther*, 15: Hodgson RJ, Rachman S, Obsessional-compulsive complaints, 389–395, 1977 with permission from Elsevier Science.
†Answers that support a diagnosis of OCD are underlined.

28. I spend a lot of time every day checking things over and over again.   *True*   False

29. Hanging and folding my clothes at night does not take up a lot of time.   True   *False*

30. Even when I do something very carefully I often feel that it is not quite right.   *True*   False

Comprehensive Psychopathological Rating Scale*
Obsessive-Compulsive Disorder Subscale Reported
Psychopathology

Name _____ Date _____ Rater _____

1. Sadness

Representing subjectively experienced mood, regardless of whether it is reflected in appearance or not. Includes depressed mood, low spirits, despondency, and the feeling of being beyond help and without hope. Rate according to intensity, duration, and the extent to which the mood is influenced by events.
Elated mood is scored 0 on this item.

    0—Occasional sadness may occur in the circumstances.

    1—Predominant feelings of sadness, but brighter moments occur.

    2—Pervasive feelings of sadness or gloominess. The mood is hardly influenced by external circumstances.

    3—Continuous experience of misery or extreme despondency.

2. Inner Tension

Representing feelings of ill-defined discomfort, edginess, inner turmoil, mental tension mounting to panic, dread, and anguish.
Rate according to intensity, frequency, duration, and the extent of reassurance called for.
Distinguish from sadness (1) and worrying (3).

    0—Placid. Only fleeting inner tension.

    1—Occasional feelings of edginess and ill-defined discomfort.

    2—Continuous feelings of inner tension or intermittent panic that the patient can only master with some difficulty.

    3—Unrelenting dread or anguish. Overwhelming panic.

*From Asberg M, Montgomery SA, Perris C, et al: A comprehensive psychopathological rating scale. *Acta Psychiatr Scand (Suppl)* 1978; 271:5–9. Used by permission. http://journals.munksgaard.dk/actapsych.

3. Worrying over Trifles

Representing apprehension and undue concern over trifles, which is difficult to stop and out of proportion to the circumstances.
Distinguish from inner tension (2), compulsive thoughts (4), and indecision (6).

    0—No particular worries.
    1—Undue concern; worrying that can be shaken off.
    2—Apprehensive and bothered about trifles or minor daily routines.
    3—Unrelenting and often painful worrying. Reassurance is ineffective.

4. Compulsive Thoughts

Representing disturbing or frightening thoughts or doubts that are experienced as silly or irrational but keep coming back against one's will.
Distinguish from worrying (3).

    0—No repetitive thoughts.
    1—Occasional compulsive thoughts that are not disturbing.
    2—Frequent disturbing compulsive thoughts.
    3—Incapacitating or obnoxious obsessions occupying one's entire mind.

5. Rituals

Representing a compulsive repeating of particular acts or rituals that are regarded as unnecessary or absurd and resisted initially but cannot be suppressed without discomfort.
The rating is based on the time spent on rituals and the degree of social incapacity.

    0—No compulsive behavior.
    1—Slight or occasional compulsive checking.
    2—Clear-cut compulsive rituals that do not interfere with social performance.
    3—Extensive rituals or checking habits that are time consuming and incapacitating.

6. Indecision

Representing vacillation and difficulty in choosing between simple alternatives.
Distinguish from worrying (3) and compulsive thoughts (4).

    0—No indecisiveness.
    1—Some vacillation but can still make a decision when necessary.
    2—Indecisiveness or vacillation that restricts or prevents actions, makes it difficult to answer simple questions or make simple choices.

3—Extreme indecisiveness even in situations where conscious deliberation is not normally required, such as whether to sit or stand, enter or stay outside.

7. Lassitude

Representing difficulty getting started or slowness in initiating and performing everyday activities.
Distinguish from indecision (6).

0—Hardly any difficulty in getting started. No sluggishness.
1—Difficulties in starting activities.
2—Difficulties in starting simple routine activities, which are carried out only with effort.
3—Complete inertia. Unable to start activity without help.

8. Concentration Difficulties

Representing difficulties in collecting one's thoughts amounting to incapacitating lack of concentration.
Rate according to intensity, frequency, and degree of incapacity produced.

0—No difficulties in concentrating.
1—Occasional difficulties in collecting one's thoughts.
2—Difficulties in concentrating and sustaining thought that interfere with reading and conversation.
3—Incapacitating lack of concentration.

NIMH Global Obsessive-Compulsive Scale*

DIRECTIONS: Choose the number (1 to 15) that best describes the present clinical state of the patient based on the guidelines below:

1–3 *Minimal within range of normal.* Mild symptoms. Person spends little time resisting them. Almost no interference in daily activity.

4–6 *Subclinical obsessive-compulsive behavior.* Mild symptoms that are noticeable to patient and observer, cause mild interference in patient's life and which he or she may resist for a minimal period of time. Easily tolerated by others.

7–9 *Clinical obsessive-compulsive behavior.* Symptoms that cause significant interference in patient's life and which he or she spends a great deal of conscious energy resisting. Requires some help from others to function in daily activity.

*From Insel TR, Murphy DL, Cohen RM, et al: *Arch Gen Psychiatry* 1983; 40:605–12. Copyrighted (1983), American Medical Association.

10–12   *Severe obsessive-compulsive behavior.* Symptoms that are crippling to the patient, interfering so that daily activity 'an active struggle.' Patient *may* spend full time resisting symptoms. Requires much help from others to function.

13–15   *Very severe obsessive-compulsive behavior.* Symptoms that completely cripple patient so that he or she requires close staff supervision over eating, sleeping, etc. Very minor decision making or minimal activity require staff support. 'Worst I've ever seen.'

Clinical Global Impairment Scale

Considering your total clinical experience with this particular problem, how mentally ill is the patient at this time? Circle one (most appropriate).
1—Normal, not at all ill
2—Borderline mentally ill
3—Mildly ill
4—Moderately ill
5—Markedly ill
6—Severely ill
7—Among the most extremely ill

Clinical Global Improvement Scale

Compared to the patient's condition at the beginning of treatment, how much has he/she changed? Circle one (most appropriate).
1—Very much improved
2—Much improved
3—Minimally improved
4—No change
5—Minimally worse
6—Much worse
7—Very much worse

Source: National Institute of Mental Health (public domain).

Appendix 2: Consumer organizations involved in OCD

Australia

Anxiety Disorders Foundation of
Australia
PO Box 6198
Shopping World, NSW 2060
Tel: +0061 (0)16 282 897

Obsessive Compulsive and Anxiety
Disorders Foundation of Victoria
(Inc)
PO Box 358
Mt Waverley
Victoria 3149
Australia

Obsessive Compulsive Disorders
Support Service
Room 318
Epworth Building
33 Pirie Street
Adelaide
SA 5000
Australia

Canada

Obsessive-Compulsive Disorder
Network (OOCDN)
PO Box 151
Etobicoke
Ontario
Canada
E-mail: oocdn@interhop.net

France

Association Francaise de
Personnes souffrant de Troubles
Obsessionnels et Compulsifs
(AFTOC)
E-mail: aftoc@mail.cpod.fr
Web: www.cpod.com/monoweb/
aftoc

Association Francaise Des Tocs et
Du Syndrome Gilles de la Tourette
24, Rue Leon Gambetta
59790 Ronchin
France

Italy

GIDOC (gruppo italiano per il
disturbo ossessivo-compulsivo)
Corso Vittorio Emanuele 76
10121 Torino
Tel/Fax: +39 011 517 5239

IDEA (istituto per la depressione
e l'ansia)
Via Statuto 8
20121 Milano
Tel: +39 02 654 126
Fax: +39 02 654 716

South Africa

OCD Association of South Africa
PO Box 87127
Houghton 2041
South Africa
Tel: +0027 (0)11 881 3678

Depression and Anxiety Support
Group
Suite 209, 2nd Floor
Benmore Gardens
Greystone Drive
Benmore 2196
South Africa
Tel: +0027 (0)11 884 1797

Mental Health Information Centre
(and MRC Unit on Anxiety
Disorders)
PO Box 19063
Tygerberg 7505
South Africa
Tel: +0027 (0)21 938 9229

South America

Asociado De Portadores De
Sindrome De Tourette
Tiques E Trastornos Obsessivo
Compulsivo
Rua Drive Ovidio Pires De Silvia
Arias
Campos
S/N Sala 4025
Sao Paolo
Brazil
Tel: +0055 11 280 9198

UK

First Steps to Freedom
7 Avon Court
School Lane
Kenilworth
CV8 2GX
Tel: +44 01926 864473

Obsessive Action
Unit 108
Aberdeen Centre
22-24 Highbury Grove
London, N5 2EA
Tel: +44 (0)20 7226 4000
Fax: +44 (0)20 7288 0828
E-mail: admin@obsessive-
action.demon.co.uk
Web: www.obsessive-
action.demon.co.uk

USA

OC Foundation, Inc
337 Notch Hill Road
North Branford, CT 06471
Tel: +1 203 315 2190
Fax: +1 203 315 2196
E-mail: info@ocfoundation.org
Web: www.ocfoundation.org

Trichotillomania Learning Center
1215 Mission St, Suite 2
Santa Cruz, CA 95060
Tel: +1 831 457 1004
Fax: +1 831 426 4383
E-mail: trichster@aol.com
Web: www.trich.org

Anxiety Disorders Association of
America
11900 Parklawn Drive, Suite 100
Rockville, MD 20852
Tel: +1 301 231 9350
Fax: +1 301 231 7392
E-mail: AnxDis@adaa.org
Web: www.adaa.org

Index

Page numbers in *italic* denote figures and tables where there is no textual reference to the material on the same page.
OCD = obsessive compulsive disorder.